MICROWAVE

COOKBOOK 2022

QUICK AND EASY RECIPES FOR SMART PEOPLE

JANE ALEXANDER

Table of Contents

Chocolate and Banana............**Errore. Il segnalibro non è definito.**

Fruit and Nut Butter Cheesecake

Serves 8–10

A continental-style cheesecake, the sort you'd find in a quality patisserie.

45 ml/3 tbsp flaked (slivered) almonds
75 g/3 oz/2/3 cup butter
175 g/6 oz/1½ cups oaten biscuit (cookie) or digestive biscuit (Graham cracker) crumbs
450 g/1 lb/2 cups curd (smooth cottage) cheese, at kitchen temperature
125 g/4 oz/½ cup caster (superfine) sugar
15 ml/1 tbsp cornflour (cornstarch)
3 eggs, at kitchen temperature, beaten
Juice of ½ fresh lime or lemon
30 ml/2 tbsp raisins

Put the almonds on a plate and toast, uncovered, on Full for 2–3 minutes. Melt the butter, uncovered, on Defrost for 2–2½ minutes. Thoroughly butter a 20 cm/8 in diameter dish and cover the base and side with the biscuit crumbs. Beat the cheese with all the remaining ingredients and stir in the almonds and melted butter. Spread evenly over the biscuit crumbs and cover loosely with kitchen paper. Cook on Defrost for 24 minutes, turning the dish four times. Remove from the microwave and leave to cool. Chill for at least 6 hours before cutting.

Preserved Ginger Cake

Serves 8

225 g/8 oz/2 cups self-raising (self-rising) flour
10 ml/2 tsp mixed (apple-pie) spice
125 g/4 oz/½ cup butter or margarine, at kitchen temperature
125 g/4 oz/½ cup light soft brown sugar
100 g/4 oz/1 cup chopped preserved ginger in syrup
2 eggs, beaten
75 ml/5 tbsp cold milk
Icing (confectioners') sugar, for dusting

Closely line a 20 cm/8 in diameter soufflé or similar straight-sided dish with clingfilm (plastic wrap), allowing it to hang very slightly over the edge. Sift the flour and spice into a bowl. Finely rub in the butter or margarine. Fork in the sugar and ginger, making sure they are evenly distributed. Stir to a soft consistency with the eggs and milk. When smoothly combined, spoon into the prepared dish and cover lightly with kitchen paper. Cook on Full for 6½–7½ minutes until the cake is well risen and beginning to shrink away from the side. Allow to stand for 15 minutes. Transfer to a wire rack by holding the clingfilm. Peel away the wrap when cold and store the cake in an airtight container. Dust with icing sugar before serving.

Serves 8

Prepare as for Preserved Ginger Cake, but add the coarsely grated peel of 1 small orange with the eggs and milk.

Honey Cake with Nuts

Serves 8–10

*A star of a cake, full of sweetness and light. It is Greek in origin,
where it is known as karithopitta. Serve it with coffee at the end of a
meal.*

For the base:

100 g/3½ oz/½ cup butter, at kitchen temperature

175 g/6 oz/¾ cup light soft brown sugar

4 eggs, at kitchen temperature

5 ml/1 tsp vanilla essence (extract)

10 ml/2 tsp bicarbonate of soda (baking soda)

10 ml/2 tsp baking powder

5 ml/1 tsp ground cinnamon

75 g/3 oz/¾ cup plain (all-purpose) flour

75 g/3 oz/¾ cup cornflour (cornstarch)

100 g/3½ oz/1 cup flaked (slivered) almonds

For the syrup:

200 ml/7 fl oz/scant 1 cup warm water

60 ml/4 tbsp dark soft brown sugar

5 cm/2 in piece cinnamon stick

5 ml/1 tsp lemon juice

150 g/5 oz/2/3 cup clear dark honey

For decoration:

60 ml/4 tbsp chopped mixed nuts

30 ml/2 tbsp clear dark honey

To make the base, closely line the base and side of an 18 cm/7 in diameter soufflé dish with clingfilm (plastic wrap), allowing it to hang very slightly over the edge. Put all the ingredients except the almonds in a food processor bowl and run the machine until smooth and evenly combined. Pulse in the almonds briefly to stop them breaking up too much. Spread the mixture into the prepared dish and cover lightly with kitchen paper. Cook on Full for 8 minutes, turning the dish twice, until the cake has risen appreciably and the top is peppered with small air pockets. Allow to stand for 5 minutes, then invert into a shallow serving dish and peel away the clingfilm.

To make the syrup, place all the ingredients in a jug and cook, uncovered, on Full for 5–6 minutes or until the mixture just begins to bubble. Watch closely in case it starts to boil over. Allow to stand for 2 minutes, then gently stir round with a wooden spoon to mix the ingredients smoothly. Spoon slowly over the cake until all the liquid is absorbed. Combine the nuts and honey in small dish. Warm through, uncovered, on Full for 1½ minutes. Spread or spoon over the top of the cake.

Gingered Honey Cake

Serves 10–12

45 ml/3 tbsp orange marmalade

225 g/8 oz/1 cup clear dark honey

2 eggs

125 ml/4 fl oz/½ cup corn or sunflower oil

150 ml/¼ pt/2/3 cup warm water

250 g/9 oz/generous 2 cups self-raising (self-rising) flour

5 ml/1 tsp bicarbonate of soda (baking soda)

3 tsp ground ginger

10 ml/2 tsp ground allspice

5 ml/1 tsp ground cinnamon

Closely line a deep 1.75 litre/3 pt/7½ cup soufflé dish with clingfilm (plastic wrap), allowing it to hang very slightly over the edge. Put the marmalade, honey, eggs, oil and water in a food processor and blend until smooth, then switch off. Sift together all the remaining ingredients and spoon into the processor bowl. Run the machine until the mixture is well combined. Spoon into the prepared dish and cover lightly with kitchen paper. Cook on Full for 10–10½ minutes until the cake is well risen and the top is covered with tiny air holes. Allow to cool almost completely in the dish, then transfer to a wire rack by holding the clingfilm. Carefully peel away the clingfilm and leave until completely cold. Store in an airtight container for 1 day before cutting.

Gingered Syrup Cake

Serves 10–12

Prepare as for Gingered Honey Cake, but substitute golden (light corn) syrup for the honey.

Traditional Gingerbread

Serves 8–10

A winter's tale of the best kind, essential for Hallowe'en and Guy Fawkes night.

175 g/6 oz/1½ cups plain (all-purpose) flour
15 ml/1 tbsp ground ginger
5 ml/1 tsp ground allspice
10 ml/2 tsp bicarbonate of soda (baking soda)
125 g/4 oz/1/3 cup golden (light corn) syrup
25 ml/1½ tbsp black treacle (molasses)
30 ml/2 tbsp dark soft brown sugar
45 ml/3 tbsp lard or white cooking fat (shortening)
1 large egg, beaten
60 ml/4 tbsp cold milk

Closely line the base and side of a 15 cm/6 in diameter soufflé dish with clingfilm (plastic wrap), allowing it to hang very slightly over the edge. Sift the flour, ginger, allspice and bicarbonate of soda into a mixing bowl. Put the syrup, treacle, sugar and fat in another bowl and heat, uncovered, on Full for 2½–3 minutes until the fat has just melted.

Stir well to blend. Mix with a fork into the dry ingredients with the egg and milk. When well combined, transfer to the prepared dish and cover lightly with kitchen paper. Cook on Full for 3–4 minutes until the gingerbread is well risen with a hint of a shine across the top. Allow to stand 10 minutes. Transfer to a wire rack by holding the clingfilm. Peel away the clingfilm and store the gingerbread in an airtight container for 1–2 days before cutting.

Orange Gingerbread

Serves 8–10

Prepare as for Traditional Gingerbread, but add the finely grated peel of 1 small orange with the egg and milk.

Coffee Apricot Torte

Serves 8

4 digestive biscuits (Graham crackers), finely crushed
225 g/8 oz/1 cup butter or margarine, at kitchen temperature
225 g/8 oz/1 cup dark soft brown sugar
4 eggs, at kitchen temperature
225 g/8 oz/2 cups self-raising (self-rising) flour
75 ml/5 tbsp coffee and chicory essence (extract)
425 g/14 oz/1 large can apricot halves, drained
300 ml/½ pt/1¼ cups double (heavy) cream
90 ml/6 tbsp flaked (slivered) almonds, toasted

Brush two shallow 20 cm/8 inch diameter dishes with melted butter, then line the bases and sides with the biscuit crumbs. Cream together the butter or margarine and sugar until light and fluffy. Beat in the eggs one at a time, adding 15 ml/1 tbsp flour with each. Fold in the remaining flour alternately with 45 ml/3 tbsp of the coffee essence. Spread equally into the prepared dishes and cover loosely with kitchen paper. Cook, one at a time, on Full for 5 minutes. Allow to cool in the dishes for 5 minutes, then invert on to a wire rack. Chop three of the

23

apricots and set aside the remainder. Whip the cream with the remaining coffee essence until thick. Take out about a quarter of the cream and stir in the chopped apricots. Use to sandwich the cakes together. Cover the top and sides with the remaining cream. Press the almonds against the side and decorate the top with the reserved apricots, cut sides down.

Rum Pineapple Torte

Serves 8

Prepare as for Coffee Apricot Torte, but omit the apricots. Flavour the cream with 30 ml/2 tbsp dark rum instead of the coffee essence (extract). Stir 2 chopped canned pineapple rings into three-quarters of the cream and use to sandwich the cakes together. Cover the top and sides with the remaining cream and decorate with halved pineapple rings. Stud with green and yellow glacé (candied) cherries, if wished.

Rich Christmas Cake

Makes 1 large family cake

*A luxurious cake, full of the splendours of Christmas and well
endowed with alcohol. Keep it plain or coat it with marzipan (almond
paste) and white icing (frosting).*

200 ml/7 fl oz/scant 1 cup sweet sherry
75 ml/5 tbsp brandy
5 ml/1 tsp mixed (apple-pie) spice
5 ml/1 tsp vanilla essence (extract)
10 ml/2 tsp dark soft brown sugar
350 g/12 oz/2 cups mixed dried fruit (fruit cake mix)
15 ml/1 tbsp chopped mixed peel
15 ml/1 tbsp red glacé (candied) cherries
50 g/2 oz/1/3 cup dried apricots
50 g/2 oz/1/3 cup chopped dates
Finely grated peel of 1 small orange
50 g/2 oz/½ cup chopped walnuts
125 g/4 oz/½ cup unsalted (sweet) butter, melted
175 g/6 oz/¾ cup dark soft brown sugar
125 g/4 oz/1 cup self-raising (self-rising) flour
3 small eggs

Put the sherry and brandy in a large mixing bowl. Cover with a plate
and cook on Full for 3–4 minutes until the mixture just begins to
bubble. Add the spice, vanilla, the 10 ml/2 tsp brown sugar, the dried

fruit, mixed peel, cherries, apricots, dates, orange peel and walnuts. Mix thoroughly. Cover with a plate and warm through on Defrost for 15 minutes, stirring four times. Leave overnight for the flavours to mature. Closely line a 20 cm/8 in diameter soufflé dish with clingfilm (plastic wrap), allowing it to hang very slightly over the edge. Stir the butter, brown sugar, flour and eggs into the cake mixture. Spoon into the prepared dish and cover loosely with kitchen paper. Cook on Defrost for 30 minutes, turning four times. Allow to stand in the microwave for 10 minutes. Cool to lukewarm, then carefully transfer to a wire rack by holding the clingfilm. Peel away the clingfilm when the cake is cold. To store, wrap in a double thickness of greaseproof (waxed) paper, then wrap again in foil. Store in a cool place for about 2 weeks before covering and icing.

Fast Simnel Cake

Makes 1 large family cake

Follow the recipe for Rich Christmas Cake and store for 2 weeks. The day before serving, cut the cake in half to make two layers. Brush both cut sides with melted apricot jam (conserve) and sandwich together with 225–300 g/8–11 oz marzipan (almond paste) rolled out to a thick round. Decorate the top with shop-bought miniature Easter eggs and chicks.

Seed Cake

Serves 8

A reminder of old times, known in Wales as shearing cake.

225 g/8 oz/2 cups self-raising (self-rising) flour

125 g/4 oz/½ cup butter or margarine

175 g/6 oz/¾ cup light soft brown sugar

Finely grated peel of 1 lemon

10–20 ml/2–4 tsp caraway seeds

10 ml/2 tsp grated nutmeg

2 eggs, beaten

150 ml/¼ pt/2/3 cup cold milk

75 ml/5 tbsp icing (confectioners') sugar, sifted

10–15 ml/2–3 tsp lemon juice

Closely line the base and side of a 20 cm/8 in diameter soufflé dish with clingfilm (plastic wrap), allowing it to hang very slightly over the edge. Sift the flour into a bowl and rub in the butter or margarine. Add the brown sugar, lemon peel, caraway seeds and nutmeg and mix in the eggs and milk with a fork to form a smooth, fairly soft batter. Transfer to the prepared dish and cover loosely with kitchen paper. Cook on Full for 7–8 minutes, turning the dish twice until the cake has risen to the top of the dish and the surface is peppered with small holes. Allow to stand for 6 minutes, then invert on to a wire rack. When completely cold, peel away the clingfilm, then turn the cake the right way up. Combine the icing sugar and lemon juice to make a thickish paste. Spread over the top of the cake.

Simple Fruit Cake

Serves 8

225 g/8 oz/2 cups self-raising (self-rising) flour
10 ml/2 tsp mixed (apple-pie) spice
125 g/4 oz/½ cup butter or margarine
125 g/4 oz/½ cup light soft brown sugar
175 g/6 oz/1 cup mixed dried fruit (fruit cake mix)
2 eggs
75 ml/5 tbsp cold milk
75 ml/5 tbsp icing (confectioners') sugar

Closely line an 18 cm/7 in diameter soufflé dish with clingfilm (plastic wrap), allowing it to hang very slightly over the edge. Sift the flour and spice into a bowl and rub in the butter or margarine. Add the sugar and dried fruit. Beat together the eggs and milk and pour into the dry ingredients, stirring to a smooth soft consistency with a fork. Spoon into the prepared dish and cover loosely with kitchen paper. Cook on Full for 6½–7 minutes until the cake is well risen and just beginning to shrink away from the side of the dish. Remove from the microwave and allow to stand for 10 minutes. Transfer to a wire rack by holding the clingfilm. When completely cold, peel away the clingfilm and dust the top with sifted icing sugar.

Date and Walnut Cake

Serves 8

Prepare as for Simple Fruit Cake, but substitute a mixture of chopped dates and walnuts for the dried fruit.

Carrot Cake

Serves 8

Once called paradise cake, this transatlantic import has been with us for a good many years and never loses its appeal.

For the cake:
3–4 carrots, cut into chunks
50 g/2 oz/½ cup walnut pieces
50 g/2 oz/½ cup packeted chopped dates, rolled in sugar
175 g/6 oz/¾ cup light soft brown sugar
2 large eggs, at kitchen temperature
175 ml/6 fl oz/¾ cup sunflower oil
5 ml/1 tsp vanilla essence (extract)
30 ml/2 tbsp cold milk
150 g/5 oz/1¼ cups plain (all-purpose) flour
5 ml/1 tsp baking powder
4 ml/¾ tsp bicarbonate of soda (baking soda)
5 ml/1 tsp mixed (apple-pie) spice

For the cream cheese frosting:
175 g/6 oz/¾ cup full-fat cream cheese, at kitchen temperature
5 ml/1 tsp vanilla essence (extract)
75 g/3 oz/½ cup icing (confectioners') sugar, sifted
15 ml/1 tbsp freshly squeezed lemon juice

To make the cake, brush a 20 cm/8 in diameter microwave ring mould with oil and line the base with non-stick parchment paper. Put the carrots and walnut pieces into a blender or food processor and run the machine until both are coarsely chopped. Transfer to a bowl and work in the dates, sugar, eggs, oil, vanilla essence and milk. Sift together the dry ingredients, then stir into the carrot mixture with a fork. Transfer to the prepared mould. Cover with clingfilm (plastic wrap) and slit it twice to allow steam to escape. Cook on Full for 6 minutes, turning three times. Allow to stand for 15 minutes, then turn out on to a wire rack. Remove the paper. Invert on to a plate when cooled completely.

To make the cream cheese frosting, beat the cheese until smooth. Add the rest of the ingredients and beat lightly until smooth. Spread thickly over the top of the cake.

Parsnip Cake

Serves 8

Prepare as for Carrot Cake, but substitute 3 small parsnips for the carrots.

Pumpkin Cake

Serves 8

Prepare as for Carrot Cake, but substitute peeled pumpkin for the carrots, allowing a medium wedge which should yield about 175 g/6 oz seeded flesh. Substitute dark soft brown sugar for light and allspice for the mixed (apple-pie) spice.

Scandinavian Cardamom Cake

Serves 8

Cardamom is much used in Scandinavian baking and this cake is a typical example of northern hemisphere exotica. Try your local ethnic food shop if you have any trouble getting the ground cardamom.

For the cake:
175 g/6 oz/1½ cups self-raising (self-rising) flour
2.5 ml/½ tsp baking powder
75 g/3 oz/2/3 cup butter or margarine, at kitchen temperature
75 g/3 oz/2/3 cup light soft brown sugar
10 ml/2 tsp ground cardamom
1 egg
Cold milk

For the topping:
30 ml/2 tbsp flaked (slivered) almonds, toasted
30 ml/2 tbsp light soft brown sugar
5 ml/1 tsp ground cinnamon

Line a deep 16.5 cm/6½ in diameter dish with clingfilm (plastic wrap), allowing it to hang very slightly over the edge. Sift the flour and baking powder into a bowl and rub in the butter or margarine finely. Add the sugar and cardamom. Beat the egg in a measuring jug and make up to 150 ml/¼ pt/2/3 cup with milk. Stir into the dry ingredients with a fork until well mixed but avoid beating. Pour into the prepared dish. Combine the topping ingredients and sprinkle over the cake. Cover with clingfilm and slit it twice to allow steam to escape. Cook on Full for 4 minutes, turning twice. Allow to stand for 10 minutes, then carefully transfer to a wire rack by holding the clingfilm. Carefully peel away the clingfilm when the cake is cold.

Fruited Tea Bread

Makes 8 slices

225 g/8 oz/11/3 cups mixed dried fruit (fruit cake mix)
100 g/3½ oz/½ cup dark soft brown sugar
30 ml/2 tbsp cold strong black tea
100 g/4 oz/1 cup self-raising (self-rising) wholemeal flour
5 ml/1 tsp ground allspice
1 egg, at kitchen temperature, beaten
8 whole almonds, blanched
30 ml/2 tbsp golden (light corn) syrup
Butter, for spreading

Closely line the base and side of a 15 cm/6 in diameter soufflé dish with clingfilm (plastic wrap), allowing it to hang very slightly over the side. Put the fruit, sugar and tea into a bowl, cover with a plate and cook on Full for 5 minutes. Stir in the flour, allspice and egg with a fork, then transfer to the prepared dish. Arrange the almonds on top. Cover loosely with kitchen paper and cook on Defrost for 8–9 minutes until the cake is well risen and beginning to shrink away from the side of the dish. Allow to stand for 10 minutes, then transfer to a wire rack by holding the clingfilm. Warm the syrup in a cup on Defrost for 1½ minutes. Peel the clingfilm off the cake and brush the top with the warmed syrup. Serve sliced and buttered.

Victoria Sandwich Cake

Serves 8

175 g/6 oz/1½ cups self-raising (self-rising) flour
175 g/6 oz/¾ cup butter or margarine, at kitchen temperature
175 g/6 oz/¾ cup caster (superfine) sugar
3 eggs, at kitchen temperature
45 ml/3 tbsp cold milk
45 ml/3 tbsp jam (conserve)
120 ml/4 fl oz/½ cup double (heavy) or whipping cream, whipped
Icing (confectioners') sugar, sifted, for dusting

Line the bases and sides of two shallow 20 cm/8 in diameter dishes with clingfilm (plastic wrap), allowing it to hang very slightly over the edge. Sift the flour on to a plate. Cream together the butter or margarine and sugar until the mixture is light and fluffy and the consistency of whipped cream. Beat in the eggs one at a time, adding 15 ml/1 tbsp flour with each. Fold in the remaining flour alternately with the milk using a large metal spoon. Spread equally into the prepared dishes. Cover loosely with kitchen paper. Cook one at a time on Full for 4 minutes. Allow to cool to lukewarm, then invert on to a wire rack. Peel away the clingfilm and leave until completely cold. Sandwich together with the jam and whipped cream and dust the top with icing sugar before serving.

Walnut Cake

Serves 8

175 g/6 oz/1½ cups self-raising (self-rising) flour
175 g/6 oz/¾ cup butter or margarine, at kitchen temperature
5 ml/1 tsp vanilla essence (extract)
175 g/6 oz/¾ cup caster (superfine) sugar
3 eggs, at kitchen temperature
50 g/2 oz/½ cup walnuts, finely chopped
45 ml/3 tbsp cold milk
2 quantities Butter Cream Icing
16 walnut halves, to decorate

Line the bases and sides of two shallow 20 cm/8 in diameter dishes with clingfilm (plastic wrap), allowing it to hang very slightly over the edge. Sift the flour on to a plate. Cream together the butter or margarine, vanilla essence and sugar until the mixture is light and fluffy and the consistency of whipped cream. Beat in the eggs one at a time, adding 15 ml/1 tbsp flour with each. Using a large metal spoon, fold in the walnuts with the remaining flour alternately with the milk. Spread equally into the prepared dishes. Cover loosely with kitchen paper. Cook one at a time on Full for 4½ minutes. Allow to cool to lukewarm, then invert on to a wire rack. Peel away the clingfilm and leave until completely cold. Sandwich together with half the icing (frosting) and top the cake with the remainder. Arrange a border of walnut halves on the top of the cake to decorate.

Carob Cake

Serves 8

Prepare as for Victoria Sandwich Cake but substitute 25 g/1 oz/¼ cup cornflour (cornstarch) and 25 g/1 oz/¼ cup carob powder for 50 g/2 oz/½ cup of the flour. Sandwich together with cream and/or canned or fresh fruit. Add 5 ml/1 tsp vanilla essence (extract) to the creamed ingredients, if wished.

Easy Chocolate Cake

Serves 8

Prepare as for Victoria Sandwich Cake, but substitute 25 g/1 oz/¼ cup cornflour (cornstarch) and 25 g/1 oz/¼ cup cocoa (unsweetened chocolate) powder for 50 g/2 oz/½ cup of the flour. Sandwich together with cream and/or chocolate spread.

Almond Cake

Serves 8

Prepare as for Victoria Sandwich Cake, but substitute 40 g/1½ oz/3 tbsp ground almonds for the same amount of flour. Flavour the creamed ingredients with 2.5–5 ml/½–1 tsp almond essence (extract). Sandwich together with smooth apricot jam (conserve) and a thin round of marzipan (almond paste).

Serves 8

Prepare as for Victoria Sandwich Cake or any of the variations. Sandwich together with cream or Butter Cream Icing (frosting) and/or jam (conserve), chocolate spread, peanut butter, orange or lemon curd, orange marmalade, canned fruit filling, honey or marzipan (almond paste). Coat the top and side with cream or Butter Cream Icing. Decorate with fresh or preserved fruits, nuts or dragees. For an even richer cake, halve each baked layer to make total of four layers before filling.

Nursery Tea Sponge Cake

Makes 6 slices

75 g/3 oz/2/3 cup caster (superfine) sugar
3 eggs, at kitchen temperature
75 g/3 oz/¾ cup plain (all-purpose) flour
90 ml/6 tbsp double (heavy) or whipping cream, whipped
45 ml/3 tbsp jam (conserve)
Caster (superfine) sugar, for sprinkling

Line the base and side of a 18 cm/7 in diameter soufflé dish with clingfilm (plastic wrap), allowing it to hang very slightly over the edge. Put the sugar in a bowl and warm, uncovered, on Defrost for 30 seconds. Add the eggs and beat until the mixture froths up and thickens to the consistency of whipped cream. Gently and lightly cut and fold in the flour using a metal spoon. Do not beat or stir. When the ingredients are well combined, transfer to the prepared dish. Cover loosely with kitchen paper and cook on Full for 4 minutes. Allow to stand for 10 minutes, then transfer to a wire rack by holding the clingfilm. When cold, peel away the clingfilm. Split in half and sandwich together with the cream and jam. Sprinkle the top with caster sugar before serving.

Lemon Sponge Cake

Makes 6 slices

Prepare as for Nursery Tea Sponge Cake, but add 10 ml/2 tsp finely grated lemon peel to the warmed egg and sugar mixture immediately before adding the flour. Sandwich together with lemon curd and thick cream.

Orange Sponge Cake

Makes 6 slices

Prepare as for Nursery Tea Sponge Cake, but add 10 ml/2 tsp finely grated orange peel to the warmed egg and sugar mixture immediately before adding the flour. Sandwich together with chocolate spread and thick cream.

Espresso Coffee Cake

Serves 8

250 g/8 oz/2 cups self-raising (self-rising) flour
15 ml/1 tbsp/2 sachets instant espresso coffee powder
125 g/4 oz/½ cup butter or margarine
125 g/4 oz/½ cup dark soft brown sugar
2 eggs, at kitchen temperature
75 ml/5 tbsp cold milk

Line the base and side of an 18 cm/7 in diameter soufflé dish with clingfilm (plastic wrap), allowing it to hang very slightly over the edge. Sift the flour and coffee powder into a bowl and rub in the butter or margarine. Add the sugar. Thoroughly beat together the eggs and milk, then mix evenly into the dry ingredients with a fork. Spoon into the prepared dish and cover loosely with kitchen paper. Cook on Full for 6½–7 minutes until the cake is well risen and just beginning to shrink away from the side of the dish. Allow to stand for 10 minutes. Transfer to a wire rack by holding the clingfilm. When completely cold, peel away the clingfilm and store the cake in an airtight container.

Orange-iced Espresso Coffee Cake

Serves 8

Make the Espresso Coffee Cake. About 2 hours before serving, make up a thick glacé icing (frosting) by mixing 175 g/6 oz/1 cup icing (confectioners') sugar with enough orange juice to form a paste-like icing. Spread over the top of the cake, then decorate with grated chocolate, chopped nuts, hundreds and thousands etc.

Espresso Coffee Cream Torte

Serves 8

Make the Espresso Coffee Cake and cut into two layers. Whip 300 ml/½ pt/1¼ cups double (heavy) cream with 60 ml/4 tbsp cold milk until thick. Sweeten with 45 ml/3 tbsp caster (superfine) sugar and flavour to taste with espresso coffee powder. Use some to sandwich the layers together, then spread the remainder thickly over the top and side of the cake. Stud the top with hazelnuts.

Raisin Cup Cakes

Makes 12

125 g/4 oz/1 cup self-raising (self-rising) flour
50 g/2 oz/¼ cup butter or margarine
50 g/2 oz/¼ cup caster (superfine) sugar
30 ml/2 tbsp raisins
1 egg
30 ml/2 tbsp cold milk
2.5 ml/½ tsp vanilla essence (extract)
Icing (confectioner's) sugar, for dusting

Sift the flour into bowl and rub in the butter or margarine finely. Add the sugar and raisins. Beat the egg with the milk and vanilla essence and stir into the dry ingredients with a fork, mixing to a soft batter without beating. Divide between 12 paper cake cases (cupcake papers) and place six at a time on the microwave turntable. Cover loosely with kitchen paper. Cook on Full for 2 minutes. Transfer to a wire rack to cool. Dust with sifted icing sugar when cold. Store in an airtight container.

Coconut Cup Cakes

Makes 12

Prepare as for Raisin Cup Cakes, but substitute 25 ml/1½ tbsp desiccated (shredded) coconut for the raisins and increase the milk to 25 ml/1½ tbsp.

Chocolate Chip Cakes

Makes 12

Prepare as for Raisin Cup Cakes, but substitute 30 ml/2 tbsp chocolate chips for the raisins.

Banana Spice Cake

Serves 8

3 large ripe bananas
175 g/6 oz/¾ cup mixture of margarine and white cooking fat
(shortening), at kitchen temperature
175 g/6 oz/¾ cup dark soft brown sugar
10 ml/2 tsp baking powder
5 ml/1 tsp ground allspice
225 g/8 oz/2 cups malted brown flour, such as granary
1 large egg, beaten
15 ml/1 tbsp chopped pecan nuts
100 g/4 oz/2/3 cup chopped dates

Closely line the base and side of a 20 cm/8 in diameter soufflé dish with clingfilm (plastic wrap), allowing it to hang very slightly over the edge. Peel the bananas and thoroughly mash in a bowl. Beat in both fats. Mix in the sugar. Toss the baking powder and allspice with the flour. Stir into the banana mixture with the egg, nuts and dates using a fork. Spread smoothly into the prepared dish. Cover loosely with kitchen paper and cook on Full for 11 minutes, turning the dish three times. Allow to stand for 10 minutes. Transfer to a wire rack by holding the clingfilm. Cool completely, then peel away the clingfilm and store the cake in an airtight container.

Banana Spice Cake with Pineapple Icing

Serves 8

Make the Banana Spice Cake. About 2 hours before serving, cover the cake with a thick glacé icing (frosting) made by sifting 175 g/6 oz/1 cup icing (confectioners') sugar into a bowl and mixing to a paste-like icing with a few drops of pineapple juice. When set, decorate with dried banana chips.

Butter Cream Icing

Makes 225 g/8 oz/1 cup

75 g/3 oz/1/3 cup butter, at kitchen temperature
175 g/6 oz/1 cup icing (confectioners') sugar, sifted
10 ml/2 tsp cold milk
5 ml/1 tsp vanilla essence (extract)
Icing (confectioners') sugar, for dusting (optional)

Beat the butter until light, then gradually beat in the sugar until light, fluffy and doubled in volume. Mix in the milk and vanilla essence and beat the icing (frosting) until smooth and thick.

Chocolate Fudge Frosting

Makes 350 g/12 oz/1½ cups

An American-style icing (frosting) which is useful for topping any plain cake.

30 ml/2 tbsp butter or margarine
60 ml/4 tbsp milk
30 ml/2 tbsp cocoa (unsweetened chocolate) powder
5 ml/1 tsp vanilla essence (extract)
300 g/10 oz/12/3 cups icing (confectioners') sugar, sifted

Put the butter or margarine, milk, cocoa and vanilla essence in a bowl. Cook, uncovered, on Defrost for 4 minutes until hot and the fat has melted. Beat in the sifted icing sugar until the frosting is smooth and quite thick. Use straight away.

Fruited Health Wedges

Makes 8

100 g/3½ oz dried apple rings
75 g/3 oz/¾ cup self-raising (self-rising) wholemeal flour
75 g/3 oz/¾ cup oatmeal
75 g/3 oz/2/3 cup margarine
75 g/3 oz/2/3 cup dark soft brown sugar
6 California prunes, chopped

Soak the apple rings in water overnight. Closely line the base and side of a shallow 18 cm/7 in diameter dish with clingfilm (plastic wrap), allowing it to hang very slightly over the edge. Put the flour and oatmeal into a bowl, add the margarine and rub in finely with the fingertips. Mix in the sugar to make a crumbly mixture. Spread half over the base of the prepared dish. Drain and chop the apple rings. Gently press with the prunes over the oatmeal mixture. Sprinkle the rest of the oatmeal mixture evenly on top. Cook, uncovered, on Full for 5½–6 minutes. Allow to cool completely in the dish. Lift out by holding the clingfilm, then peel away the clingfilm and cut into wedges. Store in an airtight container.

Fruited Health Wedges with Apricots

Makes 8

Prepare as for Fruited Health Wedges, but

substitute 6 dried apricots, well washed, for the prunes.

Shortbread

Makes 12 wedges

225 g/8 oz/1 cup unsalted (sweet) butter, at kitchen temperature
125 g/4 oz/½ cup caster (superfine) sugar, plus extra for sprinkling
350 g/12 oz/3 cups plain (all-purpose) flour

Grease and base line a 20 cm/8 in diameter deep dish. Cream together
the butter and sugar until light and fluffy, then mix in the flour until
smooth and evenly combined. Spread smoothly into the prepared dish
and prick all over with a fork. Cook, uncovered, on Defrost for 20
minutes. Remove from the microwave and sprinkle with 15 ml/1 tbsp
caster sugar. Cut into 12 wedges when still slightly warm. Carefully
transfer to a wire rack and allow to cool completely. Store in an
airtight container.

Extra Crunchy Shortbread

Makes 12 wedges

Prepare as for Shortbread, but substitute 25 g/1 oz/¼ cup semolina (cream of wheat) for 25 g/1 oz/¼ cup of the flour.

Extra Smooth Shortbread

Makes 12 wedges

Prepare as for Shortbread, but substitute 25 g/1 oz/¼ cup cornflour (cornstarch) for 25 g/1 oz/¼ cup of the flour.

Spicy Shortbread

Makes 12 wedges

Prepare as for Shortbread, but sift in 10 ml/2 tsp mixed (apple-pie) spice with the flour.

Dutch-style Shortbread

Makes 12 wedges

Prepare as for Shortbread, but substitute self-raising (self-rising) flour for the plain flour and sift 10 ml/2 tsp ground cinnamon with the flour. Before cooking, brush the top with 15–30 ml/1–2 tbsp cream, then gently press on lightly toasted flaked (slivered) almonds.

Cinnamon Balls

Makes 20

A Passover Festival speciality, a cross between a biscuit (cookie) and a cake, which seems to behave better in the microwave than it does when baked conventionally.

2 large egg whites
125 g/4 oz/½ cup caster (superfine) sugar
30 ml/2 tbsp ground cinnamon
225 g/8 oz/2 cups ground almonds
Sifted icing (confectioners') sugar

Whip the egg whites until they just begin to foam, then stir in the sugar, cinnamon and almonds. Using damp hands, roll into 20 balls. Arrange in two rings, one just inside the other, round the edge of a large flat plate. Cook, uncovered, on Full for 8 minutes, turning the plate four times. Cool to just warm, then roll in icing sugar until each one is heavily coated. Allow to cool completely and store in an airtight container.

Golden Brandy Snaps

Makes 14

Quite difficult to make conventionally, these work like a dream in the microwave.

50 g/2 oz/¼ cup butter
50 g/2 oz/1/6 cup golden (light corn) syrup
40 g/1½ oz/3 tbsp golden granulated sugar
40 g/1½ oz/1½ tbsp malted brown flour, such as granary
2.5 ml/½ tsp ground ginger
150 ml/¼ pt/2/3 cup double (heavy) or whipping cream, whipped

Put the butter in a dish and melt, uncovered, on Defrost for 2–2½ minutes. Add the syrup and sugar and stir in well. Cook, uncovered, on Full for 1 minute. Stir in the flour and ginger. Place four 5 ml/1 tsp sized spoonfuls of the mixture very well apart directly on to the microwave glass or plastic turntable. Cook on Full for 1½–1¾ minutes until the brandy snaps begin to brown and look lacy on top. Carefully lift the turntable out of the microwave and allow the biscuits (cookies) to stand for 5 minutes. Lift off each one in turn with the help of a palette knife. Roll round the handle of a large wooden spoon. Press the joins together with the fingertips and slide up to the bowl end of the spoon. Repeat with the remaining three biscuits. When they are set, remove from the handle and transfer to a wire cooling rack. Repeat until the remaining mixture is used up. Store in an airtight tin. Before eating, pipe thick cream into both ends of each brandy snap and eat the same day as they soften on standing.

Makes 14

Prepare as for Golden Brandy Snaps. Before filling with cream, arrange on a baking sheet and brush the uppermost surface with melted dark or white chocolate. Leave to set, then add the cream.

Bun Scones

Makes about 8

A cross between a bun and a scone, these are exceptionally light and make a delicious treat eaten while still warm, spread with butter and a choice of jam (conserve) or heather honey.

225 g/8 oz/2 cups wholemeal flour
5 ml/1 tsp cream of tartar
5 ml/1 tsp bicarbonate of soda (baking soda)
1.5 ml/¼ tsp salt
20 ml/4 tsp caster (superfine) sugar
25 g/1 oz/2 tbsp butter or margarine
150 ml/¼ pt/2/3 cup buttermilk, or substitute a mixture of half plain yoghurt and half skimmed milk if unavailable
Beaten egg, for brushing
Extra 5 ml/1 tsp sugar mixed with 2.5 ml/½ tsp ground cinnamon, for sprinkling

Sift together the flour, cream of tartar, bicarbonate of soda and salt into a bowl. Toss in the sugar and finely rub in the butter or margarine. Add the buttermilk (or substitute) and mix with a fork to form a fairly soft dough. Turn out on to a floured surface and knead quickly and lightly until smooth. Pat out evenly to 1 cm/½ in thick, then cut into rounds with a 5 cm/2 in biscuit (cookie) cutter. Re-roll the trimmings and continue cutting into rounds. Place round the edge of a buttered 25 cm/10 in flat plate. Brush with egg and sprinkle with the sugar and cinnamon mixture. Cook, uncovered, on Full for 4 minutes, turning the plate four times. Allow to stand for 4 minutes, then transfer to a wire rack. Eat while still warm.

Raisin Bun Scones

Makes about 8

Prepare as for Bun Scones, but add 15 ml/1 tbsp raisins with the sugar.

Breads

Any liquid used in yeasted breads must be lukewarm – not hot or cold. The best way to achieve the correct temperature is to mix half boiling liquid with half cold liquid. If it still feels hot when you dip in the second knuckle of your little finger, cool it down slightly before use. Over-hot liquid is more of a problem than too cold liquid as it can kill off the yeast and stop the bread rising.

Basic White Bread Dough

Makes 1 loaf

A speedy bread dough for those who enjoy baking but are short of time.

450 g/1 lb/4 cups strong plain (bread) flour
5 ml/1 tsp salt
1 sachet easy-blend dried yeast
30 ml/2 tbsp butter, margarine, white cooking fat (shortening) or lard
300 ml/½ pt/1¼ cups lukewarm water

Sift the flour and salt into a bowl. Warm, uncovered, on Defrost for 1 minute. Add the yeast and rub in the fat. Mix to a dough with the water. Knead on a floured surface until smooth, elastic and no longer sticky. Return to the cleaned and dried but now lightly greased bowl. Cover the bowl itself, not the dough, with clingfilm (plastic wrap) and slit it twice to allow steam to escape. Warm on Defrost for 1 minute. Rest in the microwave for 5 minutes. Repeat three or four times until the dough has doubled in size. Quickly re-knead, then use as in conventional recipes or in the microwave recipes below.

Basic Brown Bread Dough

Makes 1 loaf

Follow the recipe for Basic White Bread Dough, but in place of the strong bread (plain) flour use one of the following:

- half white and half wholemeal flour

- all wholemeal flour

- half malted wholemeal and half white flour

-

Basic Milk Bread Dough

Makes 1 loaf

Follow the recipe for Basic White Bread Dough, but in place of the water use one of the following:

- all skimmed milk

- half full-cream milk and half water

Bap Loaf

Makes 1 loaf

A soft crusted and pale loaf, eaten more in the north of Britain than the south.

Make up either the Basic White Bread Dough, Basic Brown Bread Dough or Basic Milk Bread Dough. Knead quickly and lightly after the first rising, then shape into a round about 5 cm/2 in thick. Stand on a greased and floured round flat plate. Cover with kitchen paper and warm on Defrost for 1 minute. Allow to rest for 4 minutes. Repeat three or four times until the dough has doubled in size. Sprinkle with white or brown flour. Cook, uncovered, on Full for 4 minutes. Cool on a wire rack.

Bap Rolls

Makes 16

Make up either the Basic White Bread Dough, Basic Brown Bread Dough or Basic Milk Bread Dough. Knead quickly and lightly after the first rising, then divide equally into 16 pieces. Shape into flattish rounds. Arrange eight baps round the edge of each of two greased and floured plates. Cover with kitchen paper and cook, one plate at a time, on Defrost for 1 minute, then rest for 4 minutes, and repeat three or four times until the rolls have doubled in size. Sprinkle with white or brown flour. Cook, uncovered, on Full for 4 minutes. Cool on a wire rack.

Hamburger Buns

Makes 12

Prepare as for Bap Rolls, but divide the dough into 12 pieces instead of 16. Put six buns round the edge of each of two plates and cook as directed.

Fruited Sweet Bap Rolls

Makes 16

Prepare as for Bap Rolls, but add 60 ml/4 tbsp raisins and 30 ml/2 tbsp caster (superfine) sugar to the dry ingredients before mixing in the liquid.

Cornish Splits

Makes 16

Prepare as for Bap Rolls, but do not sprinkle the tops with flour before cooking. Halve when cold and fill with thick cream or clotted cream and strawberry or raspberry jam (conserve). Dust the tops heavily with sifted icing (confectioners') sugar. Eat the same day.

Fancy Rolls

Makes 16

Make up either the Basic White Bread Dough, Basic Brown Bread Dough or Basic Milk Bread Dough. Knead quickly and lightly after the first rising, then divide equally into 16 pieces. Shape four pieces into round rolls and cut a slit across the top of each. Roll four pieces into ropes, each 20 cm/8 in long, and tie in a knot. Shape four pieces into baby Vienna loaves and make three diagonal slits on top of each. Divide each of the remaining four pieces into three, roll into narrow ropes and plait together. Arrange all the rolls on a greased and floured baking tray and leave in the warm until doubled in size. Brush the tops with egg and bake conventionally at 230°C/450°F/gas mark 8 for 15–20 minutes. Remove from the oven and transfer the rolls to a wire rack. Store in an airtight container when cold.

Rolls with Toppings

Makes 16

Prepare as for Fancy Rolls. After brushing the tops of the rolls with egg, sprinkle with any of the following: poppy seeds, toasted sesame seeds, fennel seeds, porridge oats, cracked wheat, grated hard cheese, coarse sea salt, flavoured seasoning salts.

Caraway Seed Bread

Makes 1 loaf

Make up the Basic Brown Bread Dough, adding 10-15 ml/2–3 tsp caraway seeds to the dry ingredients before mixing in the liquid. Knead lightly after the first rising, then shape into a ball. Put into a 450 ml/¾ pt/2 cup straight-sided greased round dish. Cover with kitchen paper and warm on Defrost for 1 minute. Allow to rest for 4 minutes. Repeat three or four times until the dough has doubled in size. Brush with beaten egg and sprinkle with coarse salt and/or extra caraway seeds. Cover with kitchen paper and cook on Full for 5 minutes, turning the dish once. Cook on Full for a further 2 minutes. Leave for 15 minutes, then carefully turn out on to a wire rack.

Rye Bread

Makes 1 loaf

Make up the Basic Brown Bread Dough, using half wholemeal and half rye flour. Bake as for Bap Loaf.

Oil Bread

Makes 1 loaf

Make up either the Basic White Bread Dough or Basic Brown Bread Dough, but substitute olive, walnut or hazelnut oil for the other fats. If the dough remains on the sticky side, work in a little extra flour. Cook as for Bap Loaf.

Italian Bread

Makes 1 loaf

Make up the Basic White Bread Dough, but substitute olive oil for the other fats and add 15 ml/1 tbsp red pesto and 10 ml/2 tsp sun-dried tomato purée (paste) to the dry ingredients before mixing in the liquid. Cook as for Bap Loaf, allowing an extra 30 seconds.

Spanish Bread

Makes 1 loaf

Make up the Basic White Bread Dough, but substitute olive oil for the other fats and add 30 ml/2 tbsp dried onions (in their dry state) and 12 chopped stuffed olives to the dry ingredients before mixing in the liquid. Cook as for Bap Loaf, allowing an extra 30 seconds.

Tikka Masala Bread

Makes 1 loaf

Make up the Basic White Bread Dough, but substitute melted ghee or corn oil for the other fats and add 15 ml/1 tbsp tikka spice blend and the seeds from 5 green cardamom pods to the dry ingredients before mixing in the liquid. Cook as for Bap Loaf, allowing an extra 30 seconds.

Fruited Malt Bread

Makes 2 loaves

450 g/1 lb/4 cups strong plain (bread) flour

10 ml/2 tsp salt

1 sachet easy-blend dried yeast

60 ml/4 tbsp mixed currants and raisins

60 ml/4 tbsp malt extract

15 ml/1 tbsp black treacle (molasses)

25 g/1 oz/2 tbsp butter or margarine

45 ml/3 tbsp lukewarm skimmed milk

150 ml/¼ pt/2/3 cup lukewarm water

Butter, for spreading

Sift the flour and salt into a bowl. Toss in the yeast and dried fruit. Put the malt extract, treacle and butter or margarine into a small basin. Melt, uncovered, on Defrost for 3 minutes. Add to the flour with the milk and enough water to make a soft but not sticky dough. Knead on a floured surface until smooth, elastic and no longer sticky. Divide into two equal pieces. Shape each to fit a greased 900 ml/1½ pt/3¾ cup round or rectangular dish. Cover the dishes, not the dough, with clingfilm (plastic wrap) and slit it twice to allow steam to escape. Warm together on Defrost for 1 minute. Allow to stand for 5 minutes. Repeat three or four times until the dough has doubled in size. Remove the clingfilm. Place the dishes side by side in the microwave and cook, uncovered, on Full for 2 minutes. Reverse the position of the dishes and cook for a further 2 minutes. Repeat once more. Allow to stand for 10 minutes. Invert on to a wire rack. Store in an airtight container when completely cold. Leave for 1 day before slicing and spreading with butter.

Irish Soda Bread

Makes 4 small loaves

*200 ml/7 fl oz/scant 1 cup buttermilk or 60 ml/4 tbsp each skimmed
milk and plain yoghurt*
75 ml/5 tbsp full-cream milk
350 g/12 oz/3 cups wholemeal flour
125 g/4 oz/1 cup plain (all-purpose) flour
10 ml/2 tsp bicarbonate of soda (baking soda)
5 ml/1 tsp cream of tartar
5 ml/1 tsp salt
50 g/2 oz/¼ cup butter, margarine or white cooking fat (shortening)

Thoroughly grease a 25 cm/10 in dinner plate. Mix together the
buttermilk or substitute and milk. Tip the wholemeal flour into a bowl
and sift in the plain flour, bicarbonate of soda, cream of tartar and salt.
Rub the fat in finely. Add the liquid in one go and stir to a soft dough
with a fork. Knead quickly with floured hands until smooth. Shape
into an 18 cm/7 in round. Transfer to the centre of the plate. Cut a
deepish cross on the top with the back of a knife, then dust lightly with
flour. Cover loosely with kitchen paper and cook on Full for 7
minutes. The bread will rise and spread. Allow to stand for 10 minutes.
Lift off the plate with the help of a fish slice and place on a wire rack.
Divide into four portions when cold. Store in an airtight container for
up to only 2 days as this type of bread is best eaten fresh.

Soda Bread with Bran

Makes 4 small loaves

Prepare as for Irish Soda Bread, but add 60 ml/4 tbsp coarse bran before mixing in the liquid.

To Freshen Stale Bread

Put the bread or rolls in a brown paper bag or place between the folds of a clean tea towel (dish cloth) or table napkin. Heat on Defrost until the bread feels slightly warm on the surface. Eat straight away and don't repeat with leftovers of the same bread.

Greek Pittas

Makes 4 loaves

Make up the Basic White Bread Dough. Divide into four equal pieces and knead each lightly into a ball. Roll into ovals, each 30 cm/12 in long down the centre. Dust lightly with flour. Dampen the edges with water. Fold each in half by bringing the top edge over the bottom. Press the edges well together to seal. Place on a greased and floured baking sheet. Bake straight away in a conventional oven at 230°C/450°F/gas mark 8 for 20–25 minutes until the loaves are well risen and a deep golden brown. Cool on a wire rack. Leave until just cold, then split open and eat with Greek-style dips and other foods.

Jellied Cherries in Port

Serves 6

*750 g/1½ lb canned stoned (pitted) morello cherries in light syrup,
drained and syrup reserved
15 ml/1 tbsp powdered gelatine
45 ml/3 tbsp caster (superfine) sugar
2.5 ml/½ tsp ground cinnamon
Tawny port
Double (heavy) cream, whipped, and mixed (apple-pie) spice, to
decorate*

Pour 30 ml/2 tbsp of the syrup into a large measuring jug. Stir in the gelatine and leave for 2 minutes to soften. Cover with a saucer and melt on Defrost for 2 minutes. Stir to ensure the gelatine has melted. Mix in the remaining cherry syrup, the sugar and cinnamon. Make up to 450 ml/¾ pt/2 cups with port. Cover as before and heat on Full for 2 minutes, stirring three times, until the liquid is warm and the sugar has dissolved. Transfer to a 1.25 litre/2¼ pt/5½ cup basin and allow to cool. Cover and chill until the jelly mixture is beginning to thicken and set slightly round the side of the basin. Fold in the cherries and divide between six dessert dishes. Chill until completely set. Decorate with thick cream and a dusting of mixed spice before serving.

Jellied Cherries in Cider

Serves 6

Prepare as for Jellied Cherries in Port, but substitute strong dry cider for the port and 5 ml/1 tsp grated orange peel for the cinnamon.

Mulled Pineapple

Serves 8

225 g/8 oz/1 cup caster (superfine) sugar
150 ml/¼ pt/2/3 cup cold water
1 large fresh pineapple
6 whole cloves
5 cm/2 in piece cinnamon stick
1.5 ml/¼ tsp grated nutmeg
60 ml/4 tbsp medium-dry sherry
15 ml/1 tbsp dark rum
Biscuits (cookies), to serve

Put the sugar and water in a 2.5 litre/4½ pt/11 cup dish and stir well. Cover with a large inverted plate and cook on Full for 8 minutes to make a syrup. Meanwhile, peel and core the pineapple and remove the 'eyes' with the tip of a potato peeler. Cut into slices, then cut the slices into chunks. Add to the syrup with the remaining ingredients. Cover with clingfilm (plastic wrap) and slit it twice to allow steam to escape. Cook on Full for 10 minutes, turning the dish three times. Allow to stand for 8 minutes before spooning into dishes and eating with crisp, buttery biscuits.

Mulled Sharon Fruit

Serves 8

Prepare as for Mulled Pineapple, but substitute 8 quartered sharon fruit for the pineapple. After adding to the syrup with the other ingredients, cook on Full for only 5 minutes. Flavour with brandy instead of rum.

Mulled Peaches

Serves 8

Prepare as for Mulled Pineapple, but substitute 8 large halved and stoned (pitted) peaches for the pineapple. After adding to the syrup with the other ingredients, cook on Full for only 5 minutes. Flavour with an orange liqueur instead of rum.

Pink Pears

Serves 6

450 ml/¾ pt/2 cups rosé wine
75 g/3 oz/1/3 cup caster (superfine) sugar
6 dessert pears, stalks left on
30 ml/2 tbsp cornflour (cornstarch)
45 ml/3 tbsp cold water
45 ml/3 tbsp tawny port

Pour the wine into a deep dish large enough to hold all the pears on their sides in a single layer. Add the sugar and stir in well. Cook, uncovered, on Full for 3 minutes. Meanwhile, peel the pears, taking care not to lose the stalks. Arrange on their sides in the wine and sugar mixture. Cover with clingfilm (plastic wrap) and slit it twice to allow steam to escape. Cook on Full for 4 minutes. Turn the pears over with two spoons. Cover as before and cook on Full for a further 4 minutes. Allow to stand for 5 minutes. Rearrange upright in the serving dish. To thicken the sauce, mix the cornflour smoothly with the water and stir in the port. Blend into the wine mixture. Cook, uncovered, on Full for 5 minutes, stirring briskly every minute until lightly thickened and clear. Pour over the pears and serve warm or chilled.

Christmas Pudding

Makes 2 puddings, each serving 6–8

65 g/2½ oz plain (all-purpose) flour
15 ml/1 tbsp cocoa (unsweetened chocolate) powder
10 ml/2 tsp mixed (apple-pie) spice or ground allspice
5 ml/1 tsp grated orange or tangerine peel
75 g/3 oz/1½ cups fresh brown breadcrumbs
125 g/4 oz/½ cup dark soft brown sugar
450 g/1 lb/4 cups mixed dried fruit (fruit cake mix) with peel
125 g/4 oz/1 cup shredded suet (vegetarian if preferred)
2 large eggs, at kitchen temperature
15 ml/1 tbsp black treacle (molasses)
60 ml/4 tbsp Guinness
15 ml/1 tbsp milk

Thoroughly grease two 900 ml/1½ pt/3¾ cup pudding basins. Sift the flour, cocoa and spice into a large bowl. Toss in the peel, breadcrumbs, sugar, fruit and suet. In a separate bowl, beat together the eggs, treacle, Guinness and milk. Stir into the dry ingredients with a fork to make a softish mixture. Divide equally between the prepared basins. Cover each loosely with kitchen paper. Cook, one at a time, on Full for 4 minutes. Allow to stand for 3 minutes inside the microwave. Cook each pudding on Full for a further 2 minutes. Turn out of the basins when cool. When cold, wrap with a double thickness of greaseproof (waxed) paper and freeze until needed. To serve, defrost completely, cut into portions and reheat individually on plates for 50–60 seconds.

Butter Plum Pudding

Makes 2 puddings, each serving 6–8

Prepare as for Christmas Pudding, but substitute 125 g/4 oz/½ cup melted butter for the suet.

Plum Pudding with Oil

Makes 2 puddings, each serving 6–8

Prepare as for Christmas Pudding, but substitute 75 ml/5 tbsp sunflower or corn oil for the suet. Add an extra 15 ml/1 tbsp milk.

Fruit Soufflé in Glasses

Serves 6

400 g/14 oz/1 large can any fruit filling

3 eggs, separated

90 ml/6 tbsp unbeaten whipping cream

Spoon the fruit filling into a bowl and stir in the egg yolks. Beat the whites to stiff peaks and fold lightly into the fruit mixture until thoroughly combined. Spoon the mixture equally into six stemmed wine glasses (not crystal) until half-filled. Cook in pairs on Defrost for 3 minutes. The mixture should rise to the top of each glass, but will drop slightly when removed from the oven. Make a slit in top of each with a knife. Spoon 15 ml/1 tbsp of the cream on to each. It will flow down the sides of the glasses to the bases. Serve straight away.

Almost Instant Christmas Pudding

Makes 2 puddings, each serving 8

Absolutely superb, amazingly rich-tasting, deep-toned, fruity and quick to mature so they don't have to be made weeks ahead. Canned fruit filling is the prime mover here and accounts for the unfailing success of the puddings.

225 g/8 oz/4 cups fresh white breadcrumbs
125 g/4 oz/1 cup plain (all-purpose) flour
12.5 ml/2½ tsp ground allspice
175 g/6 oz/¾ cup dark soft brown sugar
275 g/10 oz/2¼ cups finely shredded suet (vegetarian if preferred)
675 g/1½ lb/4 cups mixed dried fruit (fruit cake mix)
3 eggs, thoroughly beaten
400 g/14 oz/1 large can cherry fruit filling
30 ml/2 tbsp black treacle (molasses)
Dutch Butter Blender Cream or whipped cream, to serve.

Thoroughly grease two 900 ml/1½ pt/3¾ cup pudding basins. Place the breadcrumbs into a bowl and sift in the flour and allspice. Add the sugar, suet and dried fruit. Mix to a fairly soft mixture with the eggs, fruit filling and treacle. Divide between the prepared basins and cover each loosely with kitchen paper. Cook, one at a time, on Full for 6 minutes. Allow to stand for 5 minutes inside the microwave. Cook each pudding on Full for a further 3 minutes, turning the basin twice. Turn out of the basins when cool. When cold, wrap in greaseproof (waxed) paper and refrigerate until needed. Cut into portions and reheat as directed in the Convenience Foods table. Serve with the blender cream or whipped cream.

Ultra-fruity Christmas Pudding

Serves 8–10

An oldie from Billington's Sugar, with butter or margarine replacing sugar.

75 g/3 oz/¾ cup plain (all-purpose) flour
7.5 ml/1½ tsp ground allspice
40 g/1½ oz/¾ cup wholemeal breadcrumbs
75 g/3 oz/1/3 cup demerara sugar
75 g/3 oz/1/3 molasses sugar
125 g/4 oz/2/3 cup currants
125 g/4 oz/2/3 cup sultanas (golden raisins)
125 g/4 oz/2/3 cup dried apricots, snipped into small pieces
45 ml/3 tbsp chopped roasted hazelnuts
1 small eating (dessert) apple, peeled and grated
Finely grated peel and juice of 1 small orange
50 ml/2 fl oz/3½ tbsp cold milk
75 g/3 oz/1/3 cup butter or margarine
50 g/2 oz plain (semi-sweet) chocolate, broken into pieces
1 large egg, beaten
Brandy Sauce

Thoroughly butter a 900 ml/1½ pt/3¾ cup pudding basin. Sift the flour and spice into a large bowl. Add the breadcrumbs and sugars and toss to ensure any lumps are broken down. Mix in the dried currants, sultanas, apricots, nuts, apple and orange peel. Pour the orange juice into a jug. Add the milk, butter or margarine and the chocolate. Heat on Defrost for 2½–3 minutes until the butter and chocolate have melted. Fork into the dry ingredients with the beaten egg. Spoon into the prepared basin. Cover loosely with a round of parchment or greaseproof (waxed) paper. Cook on Full for 5 minutes, turning the basin twice. Allow to stand for 5 minutes. Cook on Full for a further 5 minutes, turning the basin twice. Allow to stand for 5 minutes before inverting on to a plate and serving with Brandy Sauce.

Plum Crumble

Serves 4

450 g/1 lb stoned (pitted) plums
125 g/4 oz/½ cup soft brown sugar
175 g/6 oz/1½ cups plain (all-purpose) wholemeal flour
125 g/4 oz/½ cup butter or margarine
75 g/3 oz/1/3 cup demerara sugar
2.5 ml/½ tsp ground allspice (optional)

Place the plums in a buttered 1 litre/1¾ pt/4¼ cup pie dish. Mix in the sugar. Tip the flour into bowl and rub in the butter or margarine finely. Add the sugar and spice and toss together. Sprinkle the mixture thickly over the fruit. Cook, uncovered, on Full for 10 minutes, turning the dish twice. Allow to stand for 5 minutes. Eat hot or warm.

Plum and Apple Crumble

Serves 4

Prepare as for Plum Crumble, but substitute 225 g/8 oz peeled and sliced apples for half the plums. Add 5 ml/1 tsp grated lemon peel to the fruit with the sugar.

Apricot Crumble

Serves 4

Prepare as for Plum Crumble, but substitute stoned (pitted) fresh apricots for the plums.

Berry Fruit Crumble with Almonds

Serves 4

Prepare as for Plum Crumble, but substitute prepared mixed berry fruits for the plums. Add 30 ml/2 tbsp toasted flaked (slivered) almonds to the crumble mixture.

Pear and Rhubarb Crumble

Serves 4

Prepare as for Plum Crumble, but substitute a mixture of peeled and chopped pears and chopped rhubarb for the plums.

Serves 4

Prepare as for Plum Crumble, but substitute a mixture of stoned (pitted) and sliced nectarines and blueberries for the plums.

Apple Betty

Serves 4–6

50 g/2 oz/¼ cup butter or margarine
125 g/4 oz/2 cups crisp breadcrumbs, bought or made from toast
175 g/6 oz/¾ cup light soft brown sugar
750 g/1½ lb cooking (tart) apples, peeled, cored and thinly sliced
30 ml/2 tbsp lemon juice
Grated zest of 1 small lemon
2.5 ml/½ tsp ground cinnamon
75 ml/5 tbsp cold water
Double (heavy) cream, whipped, or ice cream, to serve

Butter a 600 ml/1 pt/2½ cup pie dish. Melt the butter or margarine on Full for 45 seconds. Stir in the breadcrumbs and two-thirds of the sugar. Combine the apple slices, lemon juice, lemon zest, cinnamon, water and remaining sugar. Fill the prepared pie dish with alternate layers of the breadcrumb and apple mixtures, beginning and ending with breadcrumbs. Cook, uncovered, on Full for 7 minutes, turning the dish twice. Allow to stand for 5 minutes before eating with thick cream or ice cream.

Nectarine or Peach Betty

Serves 4–6

Prepare as for Apple Betty, but substitute sliced stoned (pitted) nectarines or peaches for the apples.

Middle Eastern Shred Pudding with Nuts

Serves 6

This is a fine pudding from what was once known as Arabia. The orange flower water is available from some supermarkets and pharmacies.

6 large Shredded Wheats
100 g/3½ oz/1 cup toasted pine nuts
125 g/4 oz/½ cup caster (superfine) sugar
150 ml/¼ pt/2/3 cup full-cream milk
50 g/2 oz/¼ cup butter (not margarine)
45 ml/3 tbsp orange flower water

Butter a deep 20 cm/8 in diameter dish and crumble 3 of the Shredded Wheats across the base. Combine the nuts and sugar and sprinkle evenly on top. Crush over the remaining Shredded Wheats. Heat the milk and butter in a jug, uncovered, on Full for 1½ minutes. Mix in the orange flower water. Spoon gently over the ingredients in the dish. Cook, uncovered, on Full for 6 minutes. Allow to stand for 2 minutes before serving.

Cocktail of Summer Fruits

Serves 8

225 g/8 oz/2 cups gooseberries, topped and tailed

225 g/8 oz rhubarb, chopped

30 ml/2 tbsp cold water

250 g/8 oz/1 cup caster (superfine) sugar

450 g/1 lb strawberries, sliced

125 g/4 oz raspberries

125 g/4 oz redcurrants, stalks removed

30 ml/2 tbsp Cassis or orange liqueur (optional)

Put the gooseberries and rhubarb into a deep dish with the water. Cover with clingfilm (plastic wrap) and slit it twice to allow steam to escape. Cook on Full for 6 minutes, turning the dish once. Uncover. Add the sugar and stir until dissolved. Mix in the remaining fruit. Cover when cold and chill thoroughly. Add the Cassis or liqueur, if using, just before serving.

Middle Eastern Date and Banana Compôte

Serves 6

Fresh dates, usually from Israel, are readily available in the winter.

450 g/1 lb fresh dates
450 g/1 lb bananas
Juice of ½ lemon
Juice of ½ orange
45 ml/3 tbsp orange or apricot brandy
15 ml/1 tbsp rose water
30 ml/2 tbsp demerara sugar
Sponge cake, to serve

Skin the dates and slit in half to remove the stones (pits). Place in a 1.75 litre/3 pt/7½ cup serving bowl. Peel the bananas and slice directly on to the top. Add all the remaining ingredients and toss gently to mix. Cover with clingfilm (plastic wrap) and slit it twice to allow steam to escape. Cook on Full for 6 minutes, turning the dish twice. Eat warm with sponge cake.

Mixed Dried Fruit Salad

Serves 4

*225 g/8 oz mixed dried fruits such as apple rings, apricots, peaches,
pears, prunes*
300 ml/½ pt/1¼ cups boiling water
50 g/2 oz/¼ cup granulated sugar
10 ml/2 tsp finely grated lemon peel
Thick plain yoghurt, to serve

Wash the fruit thoroughly and place in a 1.25 litre/2¼ pt/5½ cup bowl.
Stir in the water and sugar. Cover with a plate and leave to soak for 4
hours. Transfer to the microwave and cook on Full for about 20
minutes until the fruit is tender. Stir in the lemon peel and serve warm
with thick yoghurt.

Stodgy Apple and Blackberry Pudding

Serves 6

A little melted butter

275 g/10 oz/2¼ cups self-raising (self-rising) flour

150 g/5 oz/2/3 cup butter or margarine, at kitchen temperature

125 g/4 oz/½ cup soft brown sugar

2 eggs, beaten

400 g/14 oz/1 large can apple and blackberry fruit filling

45 ml/3 tbsp cold milk

Cream or custard, to serve

Brush a 1.25 litre/2¼ pt/5½ cup round soufflé dish with the melted butter. Sift the flour into a bowl and rub in the butter or margarine finely. Add the sugar and mix to a soft consistency with the eggs, fruit filling and milk, stirring briskly without beating. Spread evenly into the prepared dish. Cook, uncovered, on Full for 9 minutes, turning the dish three times. Allow to stand for 5 minutes. Turn out into a warmed shallow dish. Spoon on to plates to serve with cream or custard.

Lemony Bramble Pudding

Serves 4

A little melted butter
225g/8 oz/2 cups blackberries, crushed
Finely grated peel and juice of 1 lemon
225 g/8 oz/2 cups self-raising (self-rising) flour
125 g/4 oz/½ cup butter or margarine
100 g/3½ oz/scant ½ cup dark soft brown sugar
2 eggs, beaten
60 ml/4 tbsp cold milk
Cream, ice cream or lemon sorbet, to serve

Brush a deep 18 cm/7 in diameter dish with melted butter. Combine the blackberries with the lemon peel and juice and set aside. Sift the flour into a bowl. Rub in the butter and sugar. Mix to a softish consistency with the crushed fruit, eggs and milk. Spread smoothly into the prepared dish. Cook, uncovered, on Full for 7–8 minutes until the pudding has risen to the top of the dish and the top has no shiny patches. Allow to stand for 5 minutes during which time the pudding will drop slightly. Loosen edges with a knife and turn out on to a warmed plate. Eat warm with cream, ice cream or lemon sorbet.

Serves 4

Prepare as for Lemony Bramble Pudding, but substitute raspberries for the blackberries.

Apricot and Walnut Upside-down Pudding

Serves 8

For the pudding:
50 g/2 oz/¼ cup butter or margarine
50 g/2 oz/¼ cup light soft brown sugar
400 g/14 oz canned apricot halves in syrup, drained and syrup reserved
50 g/2 oz/½ cup walnut halves

For the topping:
225 g/8 oz/2 cups self-raising (self-rising) flour
125 g/4 oz/½ cup butter or margarine
125 g/4 oz/½ cup caster (superfine) sugar
Finely grated peel of 1 orange
2 eggs
75 ml/5 tbsp cold milk
2.5–5 ml/½–1 tsp almond essence (extract)
Coffee ice cream, to serve

To make the pudding, butter the base and sides of a deep 25 cm/10 in diameter dish. Add the butter or margarine. Melt, uncovered, on Defrost for 2 minutes. Sprinkle the brown sugar over the butter so that it almost covers the base of the dish. Arrange the apricot halves attractively on top of the sugar, cut sides facing, and intersperse them with the walnut halves.

To make the topping, sift the flour into a bowl. Finely rub in the butter or margarine. Add the sugar and orange peel and toss to combine. Thoroughly beat together the remaining ingredients, then fork into the dry ingredients until evenly mixed. Spread smoothly over the fruit and nuts. Cook, uncovered, on Full for 10 minutes. Allow to stand for 5 minutes, then turn out carefully into a shallow dish. Heat the reserved syrup on Full for 25 seconds. Serve the pudding with coffee ice cream and the warm syrup.

Bananas Foster

Serves 4

From New Orleans and named after Dick Foster, who was in charge of cleaning up the city's morals in the 1950s. Or so the story goes.

25 g/1 oz/2 tbsp butter or sunflower margarine
4 bananas
45 ml/3 tbsp dark soft brown sugar
1.5 ml/¼ tsp ground cinnamon
5 ml/1 tsp finely grated orange peel
60 ml/4 tbsp dark rum
Vanilla ice cream, to serve

Place the butter in a deep 23 cm/9 in diameter dish. Melt on Defrost for 1½ minutes. Peel the bananas, halve lengthways, then cut each half into two pieces. Arrange in the dish and sprinkle with the sugar, cinnamon and orange peel. Cover with clingfilm (plastic wrap) and slit it twice to allow steam to escape. Cook on Full for 3 minutes. Allow to stand for 1 minute. Heat the rum on Defrost until just warm. Ignite the rum with a match and pour over the uncovered bananas. Serve with rich vanilla ice cream.

Mississippi Spice Pie

Serves 8

For the flan case (pie shell):
225 g/8 oz ready-prepared shortcrust pastry (basic pie crust)
1 egg yolk

For the filling:
450 g/1 lb yellow-fleshed pink-skinned sweet potatoes, peeled and cubed
60 ml/4 tbsp boiling water
75 g/3 oz/1/3 cup caster (superfine) sugar
10 ml/2 tsp ground allspice
3 large eggs
150 ml/¼ pt/2/3 cup cold milk
30 ml/2 tbsp melted butter
Whipped cream or vanilla ice cream, to serve

To make the flan case, roll out the pastry thinly and use to line a lightly buttered 23 cm/9 in diameter fluted flan dish. Prick well all over with a fork, especially where the side joins the base. Cook, uncovered, on Full for 6 minutes, turning the dish three times. If bulges appear, gently press down with fingers protected by oven gloves. Brush all over with the egg yolk to seal holes. Cook, uncovered, on Full for a further 1 minute. Set aside.

To make the filling, put the potatoes in a 1 litre/1¾ pt/4¼ cup dish. Add the boiling water. Cover with clingfilm (plastic wrap) and slit it twice to allow steam to escape. Cook on Full for 10 minutes, turning the dish twice. Allow to stand for 5 minutes. Drain. Put into a food processor or blender and add the remaining ingredients. Work to a smooth purée. Spread evenly in the baked pastry case. Cook, uncovered, on Defrost for 20–25 minutes until the filling has set, turning the dish four times. Cool to lukewarm. Cut into portions and serve with softly whipped cream or vanilla ice cream.

Jamaica Pudding

Serves 4–5

225 g/8 oz/2 cups self-raising (self-rising) flour
125 g/4 oz/½ cup mixture white cooking fat (shortening) and
margarine
125 g/4 oz/½ cup caster (superfine) sugar
2 large eggs, beaten
50 g/2 oz/¼ cup canned crushed pineapple with syrup
15 ml/1 tbsp coffee and chicory essence (extract) or coffee liqueur
Clotted cream, to serve

Butter a 1.75 litre/3 pt/7½ cup soufflé dish. Sift the flour into a bowl and rub in the fats finely. Mix in the sugar. Mix with a fork to a soft consistency with the eggs, pineapple with syrup and coffee essence or liqueur. Spread smoothly into the dish. Cook, uncovered, on Full for 6 minutes, turning the dish once. Invert on to a serving plate and leave to stand for 5 minutes. Return to the microwave. Cook on Full for a further 1–1½ minutes. Serve with clotted cream.

Pumpkin Pie

Serves 8

Eaten in North America on the last Thursday of every November to celebrate Thanksgiving.

For the flan case (pie shell):
225 g/8 oz ready-prepared shortcrust pastry (basic pie crust)
1 egg yolk

For the filling:
½ small pumpkin or a 1.75 kg/4 lb portion, seeded
30 ml/2 tbsp black treacle (molasses)
175 g/6 oz/¾ cup light soft brown sugar
15 ml/1 tbsp cornflour (cornstarch)
10 ml/2 tsp ground allspice
150 ml/¼ pt/2/3 cup double (heavy) cream
3 eggs, beaten
Whipped cream, to serve

To make the flan case, roll out the pastry thinly and use to line a lightly buttered 23 cm/9 in diameter fluted flan dish. Prick well all over with a fork, especially where the side joins the base. Cook, uncovered, on Full for 6 minutes, turning the dish three times. If bulges appear, gently press down with fingers protected by oven gloves. Brush all over with the egg yolk to seal holes. Cook, uncovered, on Full for a further 1 minute. Set aside.

To make the filling, put the pumpkin on a plate. Cook, uncovered, on Full for 15–18 minutes until the flesh is very soft. Spoon away from the skin and leave to cool to lukewarm. Blend until smooth with the remaining ingredients. Spoon into the pastry case still in its dish. Cook, uncovered, on Full for 20–30 minutes until the filling is set, turning the dish four times. Serve warm with whipped cream. If preferred, use 425 g/15 oz/2 cups canned pumpkin instead of fresh.

Oaten Syrup Tart

Serves 6–8

An up-to-date version of treacle tart.

For the flan case (pie shell):
225 g/8 oz ready-prepared shortcrust pastry (basic pie crust)
1 egg yolk

For the filling:
125 g/4 oz/2 cups toasted muesli with fruit and nuts
75 ml/5 tbsp golden (light corn) syrup
15 ml/1 tbsp black treacle (molasses)
Whipped cream, to serve

To make the flan case, roll out the pastry thinly and use to line a lightly buttered 23 cm/9 in diameter fluted flan dish. Prick well all over with a fork, especially where the side joins the base. Cook, uncovered, on Full for 6 minutes, turning the dish three times. If bulges appear, gently press down with fingers protected by oven gloves. Brush all over with the egg yolk to seal holes. Cook, uncovered, on Full for a further 1 minute. Set aside.

To make the filling, mix together the muesli, syrup and treacle and spoon into the baked flan case. Cook, uncovered, on Full for 3 minutes. Allow to stand for 2 minutes. Cook, uncovered, on Full for a further 1 minute. Serve with cream.

Coconut Sponge Flan

Serves 8–10

For the flan case (pie shell):
225 g/8 oz ready-prepared shortcrust pastry (basic pie crust)
1 egg yolk

For the filling:
175 g/6 oz/1½ cups self-raising (self-rising) flour
75 g/3 oz/1/3 cup butter or margarine
75 g/3 oz/1/3 cup caster (superfine) sugar
75 ml/5 tbsp desiccated (shredded) coconut
2 eggs
5 ml/1 tsp vanilla essence (extract)
60 ml/4 tbsp cold milk
30 ml/2 tbsp strawberry or blackcurrant jam (conserve)

For the icing (frosting):
225 g/8 oz/11/3 cups icing (confectioners') sugar, sifted
Orange flower water

To make the flan case, roll out the pastry thinly and use to line a lightly buttered 23 cm/9 in diameter fluted flan dish. Prick well all over with a fork, especially where the side joins the base. Cook, uncovered, on Full for 6 minutes, turning the dish three times. If bulges appear, gently press down with fingers protected by oven gloves. Brush all over with the egg yolk to seal holes. Cook, uncovered, on Full for a further 1 minute. Set aside.

To make the coconut filling, sift the flour into a mixing bowl. Rub in the butter or margarine. Toss in the sugar and coconut, then mix to a soft batter with the eggs, vanilla and milk. Spread the jam over the pastry case still in its dish. Spread evenly with the coconut mixture. Cook, uncovered, on Full for 6 minutes, turning the dish four times. The flan is ready when the top looks dry and no sticky patches remain. Allow to cool completely.

To make the icing, mix the icing sugar with enough orange flower water to make thickish icing; a few teaspoonfuls should be ample. Spread over the top of the flan. Leave until set before cutting.

Easy Bakewell Tart

Serves 8–10

Prepare as for Coconut Sponge Flan, but use raspberry jam (conserve) and substitute ground almonds for the coconut.

Crumbly Mincemeat Pie

Serves 8–10

For the flan case (pie shell):
225 g/8 oz ready-prepared shortcrust pastry (basic pie crust)
1 egg yolk

For the filling:
350 g/12 oz/1 cup mincemeat

For the nut crumble:
50 g/2 oz/¼ cup butter
125 g/4 oz/1 cup self-raising (self-rising) flour, sifted
50 g/2 oz/¼ cup demerara sugar
5 ml/1 tsp ground cinnamon
60 ml/4 tbsp finely chopped walnuts

To serve:
Whipped cream, custard or ice cream

To make the flan case, roll out the pastry thinly and use to line a lightly buttered 23 cm/9 in diameter fluted flan dish. Prick well all over with a fork, especially where the side joins the base. Cook, uncovered, on Full for 6 minutes, turning the dish three times. If bulges appear, gently press down with fingers protected by oven gloves. Brush all over with the egg yolk to seal holes. Cook, uncovered, on Full for a further 1 minute. Set aside.

To make the filling, spoon the mincemeat evenly into the baked flan case.

To make the nut crumble, rub the butter into the flour, then stir in the sugar, cinnamon and walnuts. Press over the mincemeat in an even layer. Leave uncovered and cook on Full for 4 minutes, turning the pie twice. Leave to stand for 5 minutes. Cut into wedges and serve hot with whipped cream, custard or ice cream.

Bread and Butter Pudding

Serves 4

Britain's favourite pudding.

4 large slices white bread

50 g/2 oz/¼ cup butter at kitchen temperature or soft butter spread

50 g/2 oz/1/3 cup currants

50 g/2 oz/¼ cup caster (superfine) sugar

600 ml/1 pt/2½ cups cold milk

3 eggs

30 ml/2 tbsp demerara sugar

Grated nutmeg

Leave the crusts on the bread. Spread each slice with the butter, then cut into four squares. Thoroughly butter a deep 1.75 litre/3 pt/7½ cup square or oval dish. Arrange half the bread squares over the base, buttered sides up. Sprinkle with the currants and caster sugar. Cover with the remaining bread, again buttered sides up. Pour the milk into a jug or bowl. Warm, uncovered, on Full for 3 minutes. Thoroughly beat in the eggs. Slowly and gently pour over the bread. Sprinkle with the demerara sugar and nutmeg. Allow to stand for 30 minutes, loosely covered with a piece of greaseproof (waxed) paper. Cook, uncovered, on Defrost for 30 minutes. Crisp the top under a hot grill (broiler) before serving.

Lemon Curd Bread and Butter Pudding

Serves 4

Prepare as for Bread and Butter Pudding, but spread the bread with Lemon Curd instead of butter.

Baked Egg Custard

Serves 4

Superb eaten on its own, with any kind of fruit salad combination or Cocktail of Summer Fruits.

300 ml/½ pt/1¼ cups single (light) cream or full-cream milk

3 eggs

1 egg yolk

100 g/3½ oz/scant ½ cup caster (superfine) sugar

5 ml/1 tsp vanilla essence (extract)

2.5 ml/½ tsp grated nutmeg

Thoroughly butter a 1 litre/1¾ pt/4¼ cup dish. Pour the cream or milk into a jug. Heat, uncovered, on Full for 1½ minutes. Whisk in all the remaining ingredients except the nutmeg. Strain into a dish. Stand in a second 2 litre/3½ pt/8½ cup dish. Pour boiling water into the larger dish until it reaches the level of the custard in the smaller dish. Sprinkle the top of the custard with the nutmeg. Cook, uncovered, on Full for 6–8 minutes until the custard is only just set. Remove from the microwave and allow to stand for 7 minutes. Lift the dish of custard out of the larger dish and continue to stand until the centre firms up. Serve warm or cold.

Semolina Pudding

Serves 4

Nursery food but still popular with everyone.

50 g/2 oz/1/3 cup semolina (cream of wheat)
50 g/2 oz/¼ cup caster (superfine) sugar
600 ml/1 pt/2½ cups milk
10 ml/2 tsp butter or margarine

Put the semolina in a mixing bowl. Blend in the sugar and milk. Cook, uncovered, on Full for 7–8 minutes, whisking thoroughly every minute, until boiling and thickened. Stir in the butter or margarine. Transfer to serving dishes to eat.

Ground Rice Pudding

Serves 4

Prepare as for Semolina Pudding, but substitute ground rice for the semolina (cream of wheat).

Steamed Suet Treacle Pudding

Serves 4

45 ml/3 tbsp golden (light corn) syrup
125 g/4 oz/1 cup self-raising (self-rising) flour
50 g/2 oz/½ cup shredded suet (vegetarian if preferred)
50 g/2 oz/¼ cup caster (superfine) sugar
1 egg
5 ml/1 tsp vanilla essence (extract)
90 ml/6 tbsp cold milk

Thoroughly grease a 1.25 litre/2¼ pt/5½ cup pudding basin. Pour in the syrup until it covers the base. Sift the flour into a bowl and toss in the suet and sugar. Thoroughly beat together the egg, vanilla essence and milk, then fork into the dry ingredients. Spoon into the basin. Cook, uncovered, on Full for 4–4½ minutes until the pudding has risen to reach the top of the basin. Allow to stand for 2 minutes. Turn out and spoon on to four plates. Serve with any sweet dessert sauce.

Marmalade or Honey Pudding

Serves 4

Prepare as for Steamed Suet Treacle Pudding, but substitute marmalade or honey for the syrup.

Ginger Pudding

Serves 4

Prepare as for Steamed Suet Treacle Pudding, but sift 10 ml/2 tsp ground ginger in with the flour.

Jam Sponge Pudding

Serves 4

45 ml/3 tbsp raspberry jam (conserve)
175 g/6 oz/1½ cups self-raising (self-rising) flour
75 g/3 oz/1/3 cup butter or margarine
75 g/3 oz/1/3 cup caster (superfine) sugar
2 eggs
45 ml/3 tbsp cold milk
5 ml/1 tsp vanilla essence (extract)
Whipped cream or custard, to serve

Spoon the jam into a thoroughly greased 1.5 litre/2½ pt/6 cup pudding basin. Sift the flour into a bowl. Rub in the butter or margarine finely, then toss in the sugar. Thoroughly beat together the eggs, milk and vanilla essence, then fork into the dry ingredients. Spoon into the basin. Cook on Full for 7–8 minutes until the pudding has risen to the top of the basin. Allow to stand for 3 minutes. Turn out and spoon portions on to four plates. Serve with cream or custard.

Lemon Sponge Pudding

Serves 4

Prepare as for Jam Sponge Pudding, but substitute lemon curd for the jam (conserve) and add the finely grated peel of 1 small lemon to the dry ingredients.

Crêpes Suzette

Serves 4

Back in fashion after a long spell in the shadows.

8 conventionally cooked pancakes, each about 20 cm/8 in diameter
45 ml/3 tbsp butter
30 ml/2 tbsp caster (superfine) sugar
5 ml/1 tsp grated orange peel
5 ml/1 tsp grated lemon peel
Juice of 2 large oranges
30 ml/2 tbsp Grand Marnier
30 ml/2 tbsp brandy

Fold each pancake in four so that it looks like an envelope. Leave aside. Put the butter in a shallow 25 cm/10 in diameter dish. Melt on Defrost for 1½–2 minutes. Add all the remaining ingredients except the brandy and stir well. Heat on Full for 2–2½ minutes. Stir round. Add the pancakes in a single layer and baste with the butter sauce. Cook, uncovered, on Full for 3–4 minutes. Remove from the microwave. Pour the brandy into a cup and heat on Full for 15–20 seconds until tepid. Tip into a ladle and ignite with a match. Pour over the crêpes and serve when the flames have died down.

Baked Apples

For 1 apple: score a line round a large cooking (tart) apple with a sharp knife, about one-third down from the top. Remove the core with a potato peeler or apple corer, taking care not to cut through the base of the apple. Fill with sugar, dried fruit, jam (conserve) or lemon curd. Place in a dish and cook, uncovered, on Full for 3–4 minutes, turning the dish twice, until the apple has puffed up like a soufflé. Allow to stand for 2 minutes before eating.

For 2 apples: as for 1 apple, but arrange the apples side by side on the dish and cook on Full for 5 minutes.

For 3 apples: as for 1 apple, but arrange in a triangle in the dish and cook on Full for 7 minutes.

For 4 apples: as for 1 apple, but arrange in a square in the dish and cook on Full for 8–10 minutes.

Broccoli with Cheese Supreme

Serves 4–6

450 g/1 lb broccoli

60 ml/4 tbsp water

5 ml/1 tsp salt

150 ml/¼ pt/2/3 cup soured (dairy sour) cream

125 g/4 oz/1 cup Cheddar or Jarlsberg cheese, grated

1 egg

5 ml/1 tsp mild made mustard

2.5 ml/½ tsp paprika

1.5 ml/¼ tsp grated nutmeg

Wash the broccoli, separate into small florets and put into a deep 20 cm/8 in diameter dish with the water and salt. Cover with clingfilm (plastic wrap) and slit it twice to allow steam to escape. Cook on Full for 12 minutes. Drain thoroughly. Beat together the remaining ingredients and spoon over the broccoli. Cover with a plate and cook on Full for 3 minutes. Allow to stand for 2 minutes.

Guvetch

Serves 6–8

A vibrantly coloured and flavour-packed Bulgarian relation of ratatouille. Serve on its own with rice, pasta or polenta or as an accompaniment to egg, meat and poultry dishes.

450 g/1 lb French or Kenya (green) beans, topped and tailed
4 onions, very thinly sliced
3 garlic cloves, crushed
60 ml/4 tbsp olive oil
6 (bell) peppers in mixed colours, seeded and cut into strips
6 tomatoes, blanched, skinned and chopped
1 green chilli, seeded and finely chopped (optional)
10–15 ml/2–3 tsp salt
15 ml/1 tbsp caster (superfine) sugar

Cut each bean into three pieces. Put the onions and garlic in a 2.5 litre/4½ pt/11 cup dish with the oil. Stir well to mix. Cook, uncovered, on Full for 4 minutes. Thoroughly mix in all the remaining ingredients including the beans. Cover with a plate and cook on Full for 20 minutes, stirring three times. Uncover and cook on Full for a further 8–10 minutes, stirring four times, until most of the liquid has evaporated. Serve straight away or cool, cover and chill if to be eaten later.

Celery Cheese with Bacon

Serves 4

6 rashers (slices) streaky bacon
350 g/12 oz celery, diced
30 ml/2 tbsp boiling water
30 ml/2 tbsp butter or margarine
30 ml/2 tbsp plain (all-purpose) flour
300 ml/½ pt/1¼ cups warm full-cream milk
5 ml/1 tsp English made mustard
225 g/8 oz/2 cups Cheddar cheese, grated
Salt and freshly ground black pepper
Paprika
Fried (sautéed) bread, to serve

Put the bacon on a plate and cover with kitchen paper. Cook on Full for 4–4½ minutes, turning the plate once. Drain off the fat, then coarsely chop the bacon. Put the celery in a separate dish with the boiling water. Cover with a plate and cook on Full for 10 minutes, turning the dish twice. Drain and reserve the liquid. Put the butter in a 1.5 litre/2½ pt/6 cup dish. Melt, uncovered, on Defrost for 1–1½ minutes. Stir in the flour and cook on Full for 1 minute. Gradually blend in the milk. Cook, uncovered, on Full for 4–5 minutes until smoothly thickened, whisking every minute. Mix in the celery water, celery, bacon, mustard and two-thirds of the cheese. Season to taste. Transfer the mixture to a clean dish. Sprinkle the remaining cheese on top and dust with paprika. Reheat, uncovered, on Full for 2 minutes. Serve with fried bread.

Artichoke Cheese with Bacon

Serves 4

Prepare as for Celery Cheese with Bacon, but omit the celery. Put 350 g/12 oz Jerusalem artichokes in a bowl with 15 ml/1 tbsp lemon juice and 90 ml/6 tbsp boiling water. Cover with clingfilm (plastic wrap) and slit it twice to allow steam to escape. Cook on Full for 12–14 minutes until tender. Drain, reserving 45 ml/3 tbsp of the water. Add the artichokes and the water to the sauce with the mustard, bacon and cheese.

Karelian Potatoes

Serves 4

A recipe from eastern Finland for springtime potatoes.

450 g/1 lb new potatoes, washed but unpeeled
30 ml/2 tbsp boiling water
125 g/4 oz/½ cup butter, at kitchen temperature
2 hard-boiled (hard-cooked) eggs, chopped

Put the potatoes in a 900 ml/1½ pt/3¾ cup dish with the boiling water. Cover with a plate and cook on Full for 11 minutes, stirring twice. Meanwhile, beat the butter to a smooth cream and stir in the eggs. Drain the potatoes and stir in the egg mixture while the potatoes are still very hot. Serve straight away.

Dutch Potato and Gouda Casserole with Tomatoes

Serves 4

A filling and warming vegetarian casserole that can be served with cooked green vegetables or a crunchy salad.

750 g/1½ lb cooked potatoes, thickly sliced
3 large tomatoes, blanched, skinned and thinly sliced
1 large red onion, coarsely grated
30 ml/2 tbsp finely chopped parsley
175 g/6 oz/1½ cups Gouda cheese, grated
Salt and freshly ground black pepper
30 ml/2 tbsp cornflour (cornstarch)
30 ml/2 tbsp cold milk
150 ml/¼ pt/2/3 cup hot water or vegetable stock
Paprika

Fill a buttered1.5 litre/2½ pt/6 cup dish with alternate layers of potatoes, tomatoes, onion, parsley and two-thirds of the cheese, sprinkling salt and pepper between the layers. Mix the cornflour smoothly with the cold milk, then gradually whisk in the hot water or stock. Pour down the side of the dish. Sprinkle the remaining cheese on top and dust with paprika. Cover with kitchen paper and heat through on Full for 12–15 minutes. Allow to stand for 5 minutes before serving.

Buttered and Fluffed Sweet Potatoes with Cream

Serves 4

450 g/1 lb sweet pink-skinned and yellow-fleshed potatoes (not yams),
peeled and diced
60 ml/4 tbsp boiling water
45 ml/3 tbsp butter or margarine
60 ml/4 tbsp whipped cream, warmed
Salt and freshly ground black pepper

Put the potatoes in a 1.25 litre/2¼ pt/5½ cup dish. Add the water.
Cover with clingfilm (plastic wrap) and slit it twice to allow steam to
escape. Cook on Full for 10 minutes, turning the dish three times.
Allow to stand for 3 minutes. Drain and finely mash. Thoroughly beat
in the butter and cream. Season well to taste. Transfer to a serving
dish, cover with a plate and reheat on Full for 1½ –2 minutes.

Maître d'Hôtel Sweet Potatoes

Serves 4

450 g/1 lb sweet pink-skinned and yellow-fleshed potatoes (not yams),
peeled and diced
60 ml/4 tbsp boiling water
45 ml/3 tbsp butter or margarine
45 ml/3 tbsp chopped parsley

Put the potatoes in a 1.25 litre/2¼ pt/5½ cup dish. Add the water.
Cover with clingfilm (plastic wrap) and slit it twice to allow steam to
escape. Cook on Full for 10 minutes, turning the dish three times.
Allow to stand for 3 minutes, then drain. Add the butter and toss to
coat the potatoes, then sprinkle with the parsley.

Creamed Potatoes

Serves 4–6

Potatoes cooked in the microwave retain their flavour and colour and
have an excellent texture. Their nutrients are conserved because the
amount of water used for cooking is minimal. Fuel is saved and there
is no pan to wash – you can even cook the potatoes in their own
serving dish. Peel potatoes as thinly as possible to retain the vitamins.

900 g/2 lb peeled potatoes, cut into chunks
90 ml/6 tbsp boiling water
30–60 ml/2–4 tbsp butter or margarine
90 ml/6 tbsp warm milk

Salt and freshly ground black pepper

Put the potato chunks in a 1.75 litre/3 pt/7½ cup with the water. Cover with clingfilm (plastic wrap) and slit it twice to allow steam to escape. Cook on Full for 15–16 minutes, turning the dish four times, until tender. Drain if necessary, then mash finely, beating in the butter or margarine and milk alternately. Season. When light and fluffy, rough up with a fork and reheat, uncovered, on Full for 2–2½ minutes.

Creamed Potatoes with Parsley

Serves 4–6

Prepare as for Creamed Potatoes, but mix in 45–60 ml/3–4 tbsp chopped parsley with the seasoning. Reheat for an extra 30 seconds.

Creamed Potatoes with Cheese

Serves 4–6

Prepare as for Creamed Potatoes, but mix in 125 g/4 oz/1 cup grated hard cheese with the seasoning. Reheat for an extra 1½ minutes.

Hungarian Potatoes with Paprika

Serves 4

50 g/2 oz/¼ cup margarine or lard
1 large onion, finely chopped
750 g/1½ lb potatoes, cut into small chunks
45 ml/3 tbsp dried pepper flakes
10 ml/2 tsp paprika
5 ml/1 tsp salt
300 ml/½ pt/1¼ cups boiling water
60 ml/4 tbsp soured (dairy sour) cream

Put the margarine or lard in a 1.75 litre/3 pt/7½ cup dish. Heat, uncovered, on Full for 2 minutes until sizzling. Add the onion. Cook, uncovered, on Full for 2 minutes. Stir in the potatoes, pepper flakes, paprika, salt and boiling water. Cover with clingfilm (plastic wrap) and slit it twice to allow steam to escape. Cook on Full for 20 minutes, turning the dish four times. Allow to stand for 5 minutes. Spoon out on to warmed plates and top each with 15 ml/1 tbsp soured cream.

Dauphine Potatoes

Serves 6

Gratin dauphinoise – one of the French greats and an experience to be relished. Serve with a leafy salad or baked tomatoes, or as an accompaniment to meat, poultry, fish and eggs.

900 g/2 lb waxy potatoes, very thinly sliced
1–2 garlic cloves, crushed
75 ml/5 tbsp melted butter or margarine
175 g/6 oz/1½ cups Emmental or Gruyère (Swiss) cheese
Salt and freshly ground black pepper
300 ml/½ pt/1¼ cups full-cream milk
Paprika

To tenderise the potatoes, place in a large bowl and cover with boiling water. Leave for 10 minutes, then drain. Combine the garlic with the butter or margarine. Butter a deep 25 cm/10 in diameter dish. Beginning and ending with potatoes, fill the dish with alternate layers of potato slices, two-thirds of the cheese and two-thirds of the butter mixture, sprinkling salt and pepper between the layers. Pour the milk carefully down the side of the dish, then scatter over the remaining cheese and garlic butter. Sprinkle with paprika. Cover with clingfilm (plastic wrap) and slit it twice to allow steam to escape. Cook on Full for 20 minutes, turning the dish four times. The potatoes should be slightly al dente, like pasta, but if you would prefer them softer, cook on Full for an extra 3–5 minutes. Allow to stand for 5 minutes, then uncover and serve.

Savoyard Potatoes

Serves 6

Prepare as for Dauphine Potatoes, but substitute stock, or half white wine and half stock, for the milk.

Château Potatoes

Serves 6

Prepare as for Dauphine Potatoes, but substitute medium cider for the milk.

Potatoes with Almond Butter Sauce

Serves 4–5

450 g/1 lb new potatoes, unpeeled and scrubbed
30 ml/2 tbsp water
75 g/3 oz/1/3 cup unsalted (sweet) butter
75 g/3 oz/¾ cup flaked (slivered) almonds, toasted and crumbled
15 ml/1 tbsp fresh lime juice

Place the potatoes in a 1.5 litre/2½ pt/6 cup dish with the water. Cover with clingfilm (plastic wrap) and slit it twice to allow steam to escape. Cook on Full for 11–12 minutes until tender. Allow to stand while preparing the sauce. Put the butter in a measuring jug and melt, uncovered, on Defrost for 2–2½ minutes. Stir in the remaining ingredients. Toss with the drained potatoes and serve.

Mustard and Lime Tomatoes

Serves 4

A fresh zestiness makes the tomatoes attractive as a dish on the side with lamb and poultry, and also with salmon and mackerel.

4 large tomatoes, halved horizontally
Salt and freshly ground black pepper
5 ml/1 tsp finely grated lime peel
30 ml/2 tbsp wholegrain mustard
Juice of 1 lime

Stand the tomatoes, in a circle, cut sides up, round the edge of a large plate. Sprinkle with salt and pepper. Thoroughly combine the remaining ingredients and spread over the tomatoes. Cook, uncovered, on Full for 6 minutes, turning the plate three times. Allow to stand for 1 minute.

Braised Cucumber

Serves 4

1 cucumber, peeled
30 ml/2 tbsp butter or margarine, at kitchen temperature
2.5–5 ml/½–1 tsp salt
30 ml/2 tbsp finely chopped parsley or coriander (cilantro) leaves

Slice the cucumber very thinly, leave to stand for 30 minutes, then wring dry in a clean tea towel (dish cloth). Put the butter or margarine in a 1.25 litre/2¼ pt/5½ cup dish and melt, uncovered, on Defrost for 1–1½ minutes. Stir in the cucumber and salt, tossing gently until well coated with butter. Cover with a plate and cook on Full for 6 minutes, stirring twice. Uncover and stir in the parsley or coriander.

Braised Cucumber with Pernod

Serves 4

Prepare as for Braised Cucumber, but add 15 ml/1 tbsp Pernod with the cucumber.

Marrow Espagnole

Serves 4

A summer side dish to complement poultry and fish.

15 ml/1 tbsp olive oil
1 large onion, peeled and chopped
3 large tomatoes, blanched, skinned and chopped
450 g/1 lb marrow (squash), peeled and cubed
15 ml/1 tbsp marjoram or oregano, chopped
5 ml/1 tsp salt
Freshly ground black pepper

Heat the oil in a 1.75 litre/3 pt/7½ cup dish, uncovered, on Full for 1 minute. Stir in the onion and tomatoes. Cover with a plate and cook on Full for 3 minutes. Mix in all remaining ingredients, adding pepper to taste. Cover with a plate and cook on Full for 8–9 minutes until the marrow is tender. Allow to stand for 3 minutes.

Gratin of Courgettes and Tomatoes

Serves 4

3 tomatoes, blanched, skinned and coarsely chopped

4 courgettes (zucchini), topped, tailed and thinly sliced

1 onion, chopped

15 ml/1 tbsp malt or rice vinegar

30 ml/2 tbsp chopped flatleaf parsley

1 garlic clove, crushed

Salt and freshly ground black pepper

75 ml/5 tbsp Cheddar or Emmental cheese, grated

Put the tomatoes, courgettes, onion, vinegar, parsley and garlic in a deep 20 cm/8 in diameter dish. Season to taste and toss well to mix. Cover with clingfilm (plastic wrap) and slit it twice to allow steam to escape. Cook on Full for 15 minutes, turning the dish three times. Uncover and sprinkle with the cheese. Either brown conventionally under the grill (broiler) or, to save time, return to the microwave and heat on Full for 1–2 minutes until the cheese bubbles and melts.

Courgettes with Juniper Berries

Serves 4–5

8 juniper berries

30 ml/2 tbsp butter or margarine

450 g/1 lb courgettes (zucchini), topped, tailed and thinly sliced

2.5 ml/½ tsp salt

30 ml/2 tbsp finely chopped parsley

Crush the juniper berries lightly with the back of a wooden spoon. Put the butter or margarine in a deep 20 cm/8 in diameter dish. Melt, uncovered, on Defrost for 1–1½ minutes. Mix in the juniper berries, courgettes and salt and spread in an even layer to cover the base of the dish. Cover with clingfilm (plastic wrap) and slit it twice to allow steam to escape. Cook on Full for 10 minutes, turning the dish four times. Allow to stand for 2 minutes. Uncover and sprinkle with the parsley.

Buttered Chinese Leaves with Pernod

Serves 4

A cross in texture and flavour between white cabbage and firm lettuce, Chinese leaves make a highly presentable cooked vegetable and are greatly enhanced by the addition of Pernod, which adds a delicate and subtle hint of aniseed.

675 g/1½ lb Chinese leaves, shredded
50 g/2 oz/¼ cup butter or margarine
15 ml/1 tbsp Pernod
2.5–5 ml/½–1 tsp salt

Put the shredded leaves in a 2 litre/3½ pt/8½ cup dish. In a separate dish, melt the butter or margarine on Defrost for 2 minutes. Add to the cabbage with the Pernod and salt and toss gently to mix. Cover with a plate and cook on Full for 12 minutes, stirring twice. Allow to stand for 5 minutes before serving.

Chinese-style Bean Sprouts

Serves 4

450 g/1 lb fresh bean sprouts
10 ml/2 tsp dark soy sauce
5 ml/1 tsp Worcestershire sauce
5 ml/1 tsp onion salt

Toss all the ingredients together in a large mixing bowl. Transfer to a deep 20 cm/8 in diameter casserole dish (Dutch oven). Cover with a plate and cook on Full for 5 minutes. Allow to stand for 2 minutes, then stir round and serve.

Carrots with Orange

Serves 4–6

50 g/2 oz/¼ cup butter or margarine
450 g/1 lb carrots, grated
1 onion, grated
15 ml/1 tbsp fresh orange juice
5 ml/1 tsp finely grated orange peel
5 ml/1 tsp salt

Put the butter or margarine in a deep 20 cm/8 in diameter dish. Melt, uncovered, on Defrost for 1½ minutes. Stir in all the remaining ingredients and mix thoroughly. Cover with clingfilm (plastic wrap) and slit it twice to allow steam to escape. Cook on Full for 15 minutes, turning the dish twice. Allow to stand for 2–3 minutes before serving.

Braised Chicory

Serves 4

An unusual vegetable side dish that tastes faintly of asparagus. Serve with egg and poultry dishes.

4 heads chicory (Belgian endive)
30 ml/2 tbsp butter or margarine
1 vegetable stock cube
15 ml/1 tbsp boiling water
2.5 ml/½ tsp onion salt
30 ml/2 tbsp lemon juice

Trim the chicory, discarding any bruised or damaged outer leaves. Remove a cone-shaped core from the base of each to reduce bitterness. Cut the chicory into 1.5 cm/½ in thick slices and put in a 1.25 litre/2¼ pt/5½ cup casserole dish (Dutch oven). Melt the butter or margarine separately on Defrost for 1½ minutes. Pour over the chicory. Crumble the stock cube into the boiling water, then add the salt and lemon juice. Spoon over the chicory. Cover with clingfilm (plastic wrap) and slit it twice to allow steam to escape. Cook on Full for 9 minutes, turning the dish three times. Allow to stand for 1 minute before serving with the juices from the dish.

Braised Carrots with Lime

Serves 4

An intensely orange-coloured carrot dish, designed for meat stews and game.

450 g/1 lb carrots, thinly sliced
60 ml/4 tbsp boling water
30 ml/2 tbsp butter
1.5 ml/¼ tsp turmeric
5 ml/1 tsp finely grated lime peel

Place the carrots in a 1.25 litre/2¼ pt/5½ cup dish with the boiling water. Cover with clingfilm (plastic wrap) and slit it twice to allow steam to escape. Cook on Full for 9 minutes, turning the dish three times. Allow to stand for 2 minutes. Drain. Immediately toss in the butter, turmeric and lime peel. Eat straight away.

Fennel in Sherry

Serves 4

900 g/2 lb fennel
50 g/2 oz/¼ cup butter or margarine
2.5 ml/½ tsp salt
7.5 ml/1½ tsp French mustard
30 ml/2 tbsp medium-dry sherry
2.5 ml/½ tsp dried or 5 ml/1 tsp chopped fresh tarragon

Wash and dry the fennel. Discard any brown areas but leave on the 'fingers' and green fronds. Melt the butter or margarine, uncovered, on Defrost for 1½ –2 minutes. Gently beat in the remaining ingredients. Quarter each head of fennel and place in a deep 25 cm/10 in diameter dish. Coat with the butter mixture. Cover with a plate and cook on Full for 20 minutes, turning the dish four times. Allow to stand for 7 minutes before serving.

Wine-braised Leeks with Ham

Serves 4

5 narrow leeks, about 450g/1 lb in all
30 ml/2 tbsp butter or margarine, at kitchen temperature
225 g/8 oz/2 cups cooked ham, chopped
60 ml/4 tbsp red wine
Salt and freshly ground black pepper

Trim off the whiskery ends of the leeks, then cut off all but 10 cm/4 in of green 'skirt' from each. Carefully halve the leeks lengthways almost to the top. Wash thoroughly between the leaves under cold running water to remove any earth or grit. Put the butter or margarine in a 25 x 20 cm/10 x 8 in dish. Melt on Defrost for 1–1½ minutes, then brush over the base and sides. Arrange the leeks, in a single layer, over the base. Sprinkle with the ham and wine and season. Cover with clingfilm (plastic wrap) and slit it twice to allow steam to escape. Cook on Full for 15 minutes, turning the dish twice. Allow to stand for 5 minutes.

Casseroled Leeks

Serves 4

5 narrow leeks, about 450g/1 lb in all
30 ml/2 tbsp butter or margarine
60 ml/4 tbsp vegetable stock
Salt and freshly ground black pepper

Trim off the whiskery ends of the leeks, then cut off all but 10 cm/4 in of green 'skirt' from each. Carefully halve the leeks lengthways almost to the top. Wash thoroughly between the leaves under cold running water to remove any earth or grit. Cut into 1.5 cm/½ in thick slices. Place in a 1.75 litre/3 pt/7½ cup casserole dish (Dutch oven). In a separate bowl, melt the butter or margarine on Defrost for 1½ minutes. Add the stock and season well to taste. Spoon over the leeks. Cover with a plate and cook on Full for 10 minutes, stirring twice.

Casseroled Celery

Serves 4

Prepare as for Casseroled Leeks, but substitute 450 g/1 lb washed celery for the leeks. If liked, add a small chopped onion and cook for an extra 1½ minutes.

Meat-stuffed Peppers

Serves 4

4 green (bell) peppers
30 ml/2 tbsp butter or margarine
1 onion, finely chopped
225 g/8 oz/2 cups lean minced (ground) beef
30 ml/2 tbsp long-grain rice
5 ml/1 tsp dried mixed herbs
5 ml/1 tsp salt
120 ml/4 fl oz/¼ cup hot water

Cut the tops off the peppers and reserve. Discard the inside fibres and seeds from each pepper. Cut a thin sliver off each base so that they stand upright without toppling over. Put the butter or margarine in a dish and heat on Full for 1 minute. Add the onion. Cook, uncovered, on Full for 3 minutes. Mix in the meat, breaking it up with a fork. Cook, uncovered, on Full for 3 minutes. Stir in the rice, herbs, salt and 60 ml/4 tbsp of the water. Spoon the mixture into the peppers. Arrange upright and close together in a clean deep dish. Replace the lids and pour the rest of the water into the dish around the peppers for gravy. Cover with clingfilm (plastic wrap) and slit it twice to allow steam to escape. Cook on Full for 15 minutes, turning the dish twice. Allow to stand for 10 minutes before serving.

Meat-stuffed Peppers with Tomato

Serves 4

Prepare as for Meat-stuffed Peppers, but substitute tomato juice sweetened with 10 ml/2 tsp caster (superfine) sugar for the water.

Turkey-stuffed Peppers with Lemon and Thyme

Serves 4

Prepare as for Meat-stuffed Peppers, but substitute minced (ground) turkey for the beef and 2.5 ml/½ tsp thyme for the mixed herbs. Add 5 ml/1 tsp finely grated lemon peel.

Polish-style Creamed Mushrooms

Serves 6

Commonplace in Poland and Russia where mushrooms take pride of place on any table. Eat with new potatoes and boiled eggs.

30 ml/2 tbsp butter or margarine
450 g/1 lb button mushrooms
30 ml/2 tbsp cornflour (cornstarch)
30 ml/2 tbsp cold water
300 ml/½ pt/1¼ cups soured (dairy sour) cream
10 ml/2 tsp salt

Put the butter or margarine in a deep 2.25 litre/4 pt/10 cup dish. Melt, uncovered, on Defrost for 1½ minutes. Mix in the mushrooms. Cover with a plate and cook on Full for 5 minutes, stirring twice. Blend the cornflour smoothly with the water and stir in the cream. Gently stir into the mushrooms. Cover as before and cook on Full for 7–8 minutes, stirring three times, until thick and creamy. Fold in the salt and eat straight away.

Paprika Mushrooms

serves 6

Prepare as for Polish-style Creamed Mushrooms, but add 1 crushed garlic clove to the butter or margarine before melting. Mix in 15 ml/1 tbsp each tomato purée (paste) and paprika with the mushrooms. Serve with small pasta.

Curried Mushrooms

serves 6

Prepare as for Polish-style Creamed Mushrooms, but add 15–30 ml/1–2 tbsp mild curry paste and one crushed garlic clove to the butter or margarine before melting. Substitute thick plain yoghurt for the cream and fold in 10 ml/2 tsp caster (superfine) sugar with the salt. Serve with rice.

Lentil Dhal

Serves 6–7

Distinctively Oriental with its roots in India, this Lentil Dhal is graciously flavoured with a myriad spices and can be served either as an accompaniment to curries or by itself with rice as a nutritious and complete meal.

50 g/2 oz/¼ cup ghee, butter or margarine
4 onions, chopped
1–2 garlic cloves, crushed
225 g/8 oz/11/3 cups orange lentils, thoroughly rinsed
5 ml/1 tsp turmeric
5 ml/1 tsp paprika
2.5 ml/½ tsp ground ginger
20 ml/4 tsp garam masala
1.5 ml/¼ tsp cayenne pepper
Seeds from 4 green cardamom pods
15 ml/1 tbsp tomato purée (paste)
750 ml/1¼ pts/3 cups boiling water
7.5 ml/1½ tsp salt
Chopped coriander (cilantro) leaves, to garnish

Put the ghee, butter or margarine in a 1.75 litre/3 pt/7½ cup casserole dish (Dutch oven). Heat, uncovered, on Full for 1 minute. Mix in the onions and garlic. Cover with a plate and cook on Full for 3 minutes. Stir in all the remaining ingredients Cover with a plate and cook on Full for 15 minutes, stirring four times. Allow to stand for 3 minutes. If too thick for personal taste, thin down with a little extra boiling water. Fluff up with fork before serving garnished with the coriander.

Dhal with Onions and Tomatoes

Serves 6–7

3 onions
50 g/2 oz/¼ cup ghee, butter or margarine
1–2 garlic cloves, crushed
225 g/8 oz/11/3 cups orange lentils, thoroughly rinsed
3 tomatoes, blanched, skinned and chopped
5 ml/1 tsp turmeric
5 ml/1 tsp paprika
2.5 ml/½ tsp ground ginger
20 ml/4 tsp garam masala
1.5 ml/¼ tsp cayenne pepper
Seeds from 4 green cardamom pods
15 ml/1 tbsp tomato purée (paste)
750 ml/1¼ pts/3 cups boiling water
7.5 ml/1½ tsp salt
1 large onion, thinly sliced
10 ml/2 tsp sunflower or corn oil

Thinly slice 1 onion and chop the remainder. Put the ghee, butter or margarine in a 1.75 litre/3 pt/7½ cup casserole dish (Dutch oven). Heat, uncovered, on Full for 1 minute. Mix in the chopped onions and garlic. Cover with a plate and cook on Full for 3 minutes. Stir in all the remaining ingredients. Cover with a plate and cook on Full for 15 minutes, stirring four times. Allow to stand for 3 minutes. If too thick for personal taste, thin down with a little extra boiling water. Separate the sliced onion into rings and fry (sauté) conventionally in the oil until lightly golden and crisp. Fluff up the dhal with a fork before serving garnished with the onion rings. (Alternatively, omit the sliced onion and instead garnish with ready-prepared fried onions available from supermarkets.)

Vegetable Madras

Serves 4

25 g/1 oz/2 tbsp ghee or 15 ml/1 tbsp groundnut (peanut) oil

1 onion, peeled and chopped

1 leek, trimmed and chopped

2 garlic cloves, crushed

15 ml/1 tbsp hot curry powder

5 ml/1 tsp ground cumin

5 ml/1 tsp garam masala

2.5 ml/½ tsp turmeric

Juice of 1 small lemon

150 ml/¼ pt/2/3 cup vegetable stock

30 ml/2 tbsp tomato purée (paste)

30 ml/2 tbsp toasted cashew nuts

450 g/1 lb mixed cooked root vegetables, diced

175 g/6 oz/¾ cup brown rice, boiled

Popadoms, to serve

Put the ghee or oil in a 2.5 litre/4½ pt/11 cup dish. Heat, uncovered, on Full for 1 minute. Add the onion, leek and garlic and mix in thoroughly. Cook, uncovered, on Full for 3 minutes. Add the curry powder, cumin, garam masala, turmeric and lemon juice. Cook, uncovered, on Full for 3 minutes, stirring twice. Add the stock, tomato purée and cashew nuts. Cover with an inverted plate and cook on Full for 5 minutes. Stir in the vegetables. Cover as before and heat through on Full for 4 minutes. Serve with the brown rice and popadoms.

Mixed Vegetable Curry

Serves 6

1.6 kg/3½ lb mixed vegetables, such as red or green (bell) peppers;

courgettes (zucchini); unpeeled aubergines (eggplants); carrots;

potatoes; Brussels sprouts or broccoli; onions; leeks

30 ml/2 tbsp groundnut (peanut) or corn oil

2 garlic cloves, crushed

60 ml/4 tbsp tomato purée (paste)

45 ml/3 tbsp garam masala

30 ml/2 tbsp mild, medium or hot curry powder

5 ml/1 tsp ground coriander (cilantro)

5 ml/1 tsp ground cumin

15 ml/1 tbsp salt

1 large bay leaf

400 g/14 oz/1 large can chopped tomatoes

15 ml/1 tbsp caster (superfine) sugar

150 ml/¼ pt/2/3 cup boiling water

250 g/9 oz/generous 1 cup basmati or long-grain rice, boiled

Thick plain yoghurt, to serve

Prepare all the vegetables according to type. Cut into small cubes or slice where appropriate. Place in a 2.75 litre/5 pt/12 cup deep dish. Mix in all the remaining ingredients except the boiling water and rice. Cover with a large plate and cook on Full for 25–30 minutes, stirring four times, until the vegetables are tender but still firm to the bite. Remove the bay leaf, blend in the water and adjust the seasonings to taste – the curry may need some extra salt. Serve with the rice and a bowl of thick plain yoghurt.

Jellied Mediterranean Salad

Serves 6

300 ml/½ pt/1¼ cups cold vegetable stock or vegetable cooking water
15 ml/1 tbsp powdered gelatine
45 ml/3 tbsp tomato juice
45 ml/3 tbsp red wine
1 green (bell) pepper, seeded and cut into strips
2 tomatoes, blanched, skinned and chopped
30 ml/2 tbsp drained capers
50g /2 oz/¼ cup chopped gherkins (cornichons)
12 stuffed olives, sliced
10 ml/2 tsp anchovy sauce

Pour 45 ml/3 tbsp of the stock or vegetable cooking water in a bowl.
Stir in the gelatine. Allow to stand for 5 minutes to soften. Melt,
uncovered, on Defrost for 2–2½ minutes. Stir in the remaining stock
with the tomato juice and wine. Cover when cold, then chill until just
beginning to thicken and set. Place the pepper strips in a bowl and
cover with boiling water. Leave for 5 minutes to soften, then drain.
Stir the tomatoes and pepper strips into the setting jelly with all the
remaining ingredients. Transfer to a 1.25 litre/2¼ pt/5½ cup wetted
jelly mould or basin. Cover and chill for several hours until firm. To
serve, dip the mould or basin in and out of bowl of hot water to loosen,
then run a hot wet knife gently round the sides. Invert on to a wetted
plate before serving. (The wetting stops the jelly sticking.)

Jellied Greek Salad

Serves 6

Prepare as for Jellied Mediterranean Salad, but omit the capers and gherkins (cornichons). Add 125 g/4 oz/1 cup finely diced Feta cheese and 1 small chopped onion. Substitute stoned (pitted) black olives for stuffed.

Jellied Russian Salad

Serves 6

Prepare as for Jellied Mediterranean Salad, but substitute 90 ml/6 tbsp mayonnaise for the tomato juice and wine and 225 g/8 oz/2 cups diced carrots and potatoes for the tomatoes and (bell) pepper. Add 30 ml/2 tbsp cooked peas.

Kohlrabi Salad with Mustardy Mayonnaise

Serves 6

900 g/2 lb kohlrabi
75 ml/5 tbsp boiling water
5 ml/1 tsp salt
10 ml/2 tsp lemon juice
60–120 ml/4–6 tbsp thick mayonnaise
10–20 ml/2–4 tsp wholegrain mustard
Sliced radishes, to garnish

Peel the kohlrabi thickly, wash well and cut each head into eight pieces Place in a 1.25 litre/3 pt/7½ cup dish with the water, salt and lemon juice. Cover with clingfilm (plastic wrap) and slit it twice to allow steam to escape. Cook on Full for 10–15 minutes, turning the dish three times, until tender. Drain and slice or dice and put in a mixing bowl. Mix together the mayonnaise and mustard and toss the kohlrabi in this mixture until the pieces are thoroughly coated. Transfer to a serving dish and garnish with the radish slices.

Beetroot, Celery and Apple Cups

Serves 6

60 ml/4 tbsp cold water

15 ml/1 tbsp powdered gelatine

225 ml/8 fl oz/1 cup apple juice

30 ml/2 tbsp raspberry vinegar

5 ml/1 tsp salt

225 g/8 oz cooked (not pickled) beetroot (red beets), coarsely grated

1 eating (dessert) apple, peeled and coarsely grated

1 celery stalk, cut into thin matchsticks

1 small onion, chopped

Pour 45 ml/3 tbsp of the cold water in a small bowl and stir in the gelatine. Leave to stand for 5 minutes to soften. Melt, uncovered, on Defrost for 2–2½ minutes. Stir in the remaining cold water with the apple juice, vinegar and salt. Cover when cold, then chill until just beginning to thicken and set. Add the beetroot, apple, celery and onion to the part-set jelly and stir gently until thoroughly combined. Transfer to six small wetted cups, then cover and chill until firm and set. Turn out on to individual plates.

Mock Waldorf Cups

Serves 6

Prepare as for Beetroot, Celery and Apple Cups, but add 30 ml/2 tbsp chopped walnuts with the vegetables and apple.

Celeriac Salad with Garlic, Mayonnaise and Pistachios

Serves 6

900 g/2 lb celeriac (celery root)
300 ml/½ pt/1¼ cups cold water
15 ml/1 tbsp lemon juice
7.5 ml/1½ tsp salt
1 garlic clove, crushed
45 ml/3 tbsp coarsely chopped pistachio nuts
60–120 ml/4–8 tbsp thick mayonnaise
Radicchio leaves and whole pistachio nuts, to garnish

Peel the celeriac thickly, wash well and cut each head into eight pieces. Place in a 2.25 litre/4 pt/10 cup dish with the water, lemon juice and salt. Cover with clingfilm (plastic wrap) and slit it twice to allow steam to escape. Cook on Full for 20 minutes, turning the dish four times. Drain and slice and put in a mixing bowl. Add the garlic and chopped pistachio nuts. While still warm, toss with the mayonnaise until the pieces of celeriac are thoroughly coated. Transfer to a serving dish. Garnish with radicchio leaves and pistachios before serving, if possible while still slightly warm.

Continental Celeriac Salad

Serves 4

An assembly of fine and complementary flavours makes this a suitable Christmas salad to go with cold turkey and gammon.

750 g/1½ lb celeriac (celery root)
75 ml/5 tbsp boiling water
5 ml/1 tsp salt
10 ml/2 tsp lemon juice
For the dressing:
30 ml/2 tbsp corn or sunflower oil
15 ml/1 tbsp malt or cider vinegar
15 ml/1 tbsp made mustard
2.5–5 ml/½–1 tsp caraway seeds
1.5 ml/¼ tsp tsp salt
5 ml/1 tsp caster (superfine) sugar
Freshly ground black pepper

Peel the celeriac thickly and cut it into small cubes. Place in a 1.75 litre/3 pt/7½ cup dish. Add the boiling water, salt and lemon juice. Cover with clingfilm (plastic wrap) and slit it twice to allow steam to escape. Cook on Full for 10–15 minutes, turning the dish three times, until tender. Drain. Thoroughly beat together all the remaining ingredients. Add to the hot celeriac and toss thoroughly. Cover and allow to cool. Serve at room temperature.

Serves 4

Prepare as for Continental Celeriac Salad, but add 4 rashers (slices) bacon, crisply grilled (broiled) and crumbled, at the same time as the dressing.

Artichoke Salad with Peppers and Eggs in Warm Dressing

Serves 6

400 g/14 oz/1 large can artichoke hearts, drained

400 g/14 oz/1 large can red pimientos, drained

10 ml/2 tsp red wine vinegar

60 ml/4 tbsp lemon juice

125 ml/4 fl oz/½ cup olive oil

1 garlic clove, crushed

5 ml/1 tsp continental mustard

5 ml/1 tsp salt

5 ml/1 tsp caster (superfine) sugar

4 large hard-boiled (hard-cooked) eggs, shelled and grated

225 g/8 oz/2 cups Feta cheese, diced

Halve the artichokes and cut the pimientos into strips. Arrange alternately round a large plate, leaving a hollow in the centre. Put the vinegar, lemon juice, oil, garlic, mustard, salt and sugar in small bowl. Heat, uncovered, on Full for 1 minute, beating twice. Pile the eggs and cheese in a mound in the centre of the salad and gently spoon over the warm dresssing.

Sage and Onion Stuffing

Makes 225–275 g/8–10 oz/11/3–12/3 cups

For pork.

25 g/1 oz/2 tbsp butter or margarine

2 onions, pre-boiled (see table page 45), chopped

125 g/4 oz/2 cups white or brown breadcrumbs

5 ml/1 tsp dried sage

A little water or milk

Salt and freshly ground black pepper

Put the butter or margarine in a 1 litre/1¾ pt/4¼ cup dish. Heat, uncovered, on Full for 1 minute. Stir in the onions. Cook, uncovered, on Full for 3 minutes, stirring every minute. Mix in the breadcrumbs and sage and sufficient water or milk to bind to a crumbly consistency. Season to taste. Use when cold.

Celery and Pesto Stuffing

Makes 225–275 g/8–10 oz/1 1/3–1 2/3 cups

For fish and poultry.

Prepare as for Sage and Onion Stuffing, but substitute 2 finely chopped celery stalks for the onions. Before seasoning, stir in 10 ml/2 tsp green pesto.

Leek and Tomato Stuffing

Makes 225–275 g/8–10 oz/1 1/3–1 2/3 cups

For meat and poultry.

25 g/1 oz/2 tbsp butter or margarine
2 leeks, white part only, cut into very thin slices
2 tomatoes, blanched, skinned and chopped
125 g/4 oz/2 cups fresh white breadcrumbs
Salt and freshly ground black pepper
Chicken stock, if necessary

Put the butter or margarine in a 1 litre/1¾ pt/4¼ cup dish. Heat, uncovered, on Full for 1 minute. Stir in the leeks. Cook, uncovered, on Full for 3 minutes, stirring three times. Mix in the tomatoes and breadcrumbs and season to taste. Bind with stock if necessary. Use when cold.

Bacon Stuffing

Makes 225–275 g/8–10 oz/11/3–12/3 cups

For meat, poultry and strong-tasting fish.

4 rashers (slices) streaky bacon, chopped into small pieces

25 g/1 oz/2 tbsp butter, margarine or lard

125 g/4 oz/2 cups fresh white breadcrumbs

5 ml/1 tsp Worcestershire sauce

5 ml/1 tsp made mustard

2.5 ml/½ tsp dried mixed herbs

Salt and freshly ground black pepper

Milk, if necessary

Put the bacon in a 1 litre/1¾ pt/4¼ cup dish with the butter, margarine or lard. Cook, uncovered, on Full for 2 minutes, stirring once. Mix in the breadcrumbs, Worcestershire sauce, mustard and herbs and season to taste. Bind with milk if necessary.

Bacon and Apricot Stuffing

Makes 225–275 g/8–10 oz/11/3–12/3 cups

For poultry and game

Prepare as for Bacon Stuffing, but add 6 well-washed and coarsely chopped apricot halves with the herbs.

Mushroom, Lemon and Thyme Stuffing

Makes 225–275 g/8–10 oz/11/3–12/3 cups

For poultry.

25 g/1 oz/2 tbsp butter or margarine
125 g/4 oz button mushrooms, sliced
5 ml/1 tsp finely grated lemon peel
2.5 ml/½ tsp dried thyme
1 garlic clove, crushed
125 g/4 oz/2 cups fresh white breadcrumbs
Salt and freshly ground black pepper
Milk, if necessary

Put the butter or margarine in a 1 litre/1¾ pt/4¼ cup dish. Heat, uncovered, on Full for 1 minute. Stir in the mushrooms. Cook, uncovered, on Full for 3 minutes, stirring twice. Mix in the lemon peel, thyme, garlic and breadcrumbs and season to taste. Bind with milk only if the stuffing remains on the dry side. Use when cold.

Mushroom and Leek Stuffing

Makes 225–275 g/8–10 oz/11/3–12/3 cups

For poultry, vegetables and fish.

25 g/1 oz/2 tbsp butter or margarine

1 leek, white part only, very thinly sliced

125 g/4 oz mushrooms, sliced

125 g/4 oz/2 cups fresh brown breadcrumbs

30 ml/2 tbsp chopped parsley

Salt and freshly ground black pepper

Milk, if necessary

Put the butter or margarine in a 1.25 litre/2¼ pt/5½ cup dish. Heat, uncovered, on Full for 1 minute. Stir in the leek. Cook, uncovered, on Full for 2 minutes, stirring once. Mix in the mushrooms. Cook, uncovered, on Full for 2 minutes, stirring twice. Mix in the breadcrumbs and parsley and season to taste. Bind with milk only if the stuffing remains on the dry side. Use when cold.

Ham and Pineapple Stuffing

Makes 225–275 g/8–10 oz/11/3–12/3 cups

For poultry.

25 g/1 oz/2 tbsp butter or margarine
1 onion, finely chopped
1 fresh pineapple ring, skin removed and flesh chopped
75 g/3 oz/¾ cup cooked ham, chopped
125 g/4 oz/2 cups fresh white breadcrumbs
Salt and freshly ground black pepper

Put the butter or margarine in a 1 litre/1¾ pt/4¼ cup dish. Heat, uncovered, on Full for 1 minute. Stir in the onion. Cook, uncovered, on Full for 2 minutes, stirring once. Mix in the pineapple and ham. Cook, uncovered, on Full for 2 minutes, stirring twice. Fork in the breadcrumbs and season to taste. Use when cold.

Asian Mushroom and Cashew Nut Stuffing

Makes 225–275 g/8–10 oz/1 1/3–1 2/3 cups

For poultry and fish.

25 g/1 oz/2 tbsp butter or margarine

6 spring onions (scallions), chopped

125 g/4 oz mushrooms, sliced

125 g/4 oz/2 cups fresh brown breadcrumbs

45 ml/3 tbsp cashew nuts, toasted

30 ml/2 tbsp coriander (cilantro) leaves

Salt and freshly ground black pepper

Soy sauce, if necessary

Put the butter or margarine in a 1.25 litre/2¼ pt/5½ cup dish. Heat, uncovered, on Full for 1 minute. Stir in the onions. Cook, uncovered, on Full for 2 minutes, stirring once. Mix in the mushrooms. Cook, uncovered, on Full for 2 minutes, stirring twice. Mix in the breadcrumbs, cashew nuts and coriander and season to taste. Bind with soy sauce only if the stuffing remains on the dry side. Use when cold.

Ham and Carrot Stuffing

Makes 225–275 g/8–10 oz/11/3–12/3 cups

For poultry, lamb and game.

Prepare as for Ham and Pineapple Stuffing, but substitute 2 grated carrots for the pineapple.

Ham, Banana and Sweetcorn Stuffing

Makes 225–275 g/8–10 oz/11/3–12/3 cups

For poultry.

Prepare as for Ham and Pineapple Stuffing, but substitute 1 small coarsely mashed banana for the pineapple. Add 30 ml/2 tbsp sweetcorn (corn) with the breadcrumbs.

Italian Stuffing

Makes 225–275 g/8–10 oz/11/3–12/3 cups

For lamb, poultry and fish.

30 ml/2 tbsp olive oil

1 garlic clove

1 celery stalk, finely chopped

2 tomatoes, blanched, skinned and coarsely chopped

12 stoned (pitted) black olives, halved

10 ml/2 tsp chopped basil leaves

125 g/4 oz/2 cups fresh crumbs made from Italian bread such as ciabatta

Salt and freshly ground black pepper

Put the olive oil in a 1 litre/1¾ pt/4¼ cup dish. Heat, uncovered, on Full for 1 minute. Stir in the garlic and celery. Cook, uncovered, on Full for 2½ minutes, stirring once. Mix in all the remaining ingredients. Use when cold.

Spanish Stuffing

Makes 225–275 g/8–10 oz/11/3–12/3 cups

For strong fish and poultry.

Prepare as for Italian Stuffing, but substitute halved stuffed olives for the stoned (pitted) black olives. Use ordinary white breadcrumbs instead of crumbs from Italian bread and add 30 ml/2 tbsp flaked (slivered) and toasted almonds.

Orange and Coriander Stuffing

Makes 175 G/6 Oz/1 cup

For meat and poultry.

25 g/1 oz/2 tbsp butter or margarine
1 small onion, finely chopped
125 g/4 oz/2 cups fresh white breadcrumbs
Finely grated peel and juice of 1 orange
45 ml/3 tbsp finely chopped coriander (cilantro) leaves
Salt and freshly ground black pepper
Milk, if necessary

Put the butter or margarine in a 1 litre/1¾ pt/4¼ cup dish. Heat, uncovered, on Full for 1 minute. Stir in the onion. Cook, uncovered, on Full for 3 minutes, stirring once. Mix in the crumbs, orange peel and juice and the coriander (cilantro) and season to taste. Bind with milk only if the stuffing remains on the dry side. Use when cold.

Lime and Coriander Stuffing

Makes 175 g/6 oz/1 cup

For fish.

Prepare as for Orange and Coriander Stuffing, but substitute the grated peel and juice of 1 lime for the orange.

Orange and Apricot Stuffing

Makes 275 g/10 oz/12/3 cups

For rich meats and poultry.

125 g/4 oz dried apricots, washed
Warm black tea
25 g/1 oz/2 tbsp butter or margarine
1 small onion, chopped
5 ml/1 tsp finely grated orange peel
Juice of 1 orange
125 g/4 oz/2 cups fresh white breadcrumbs
Salt and freshly ground black pepper

Soak the apricots in warm tea for at least 2 hours. Drain and snip into small pieces with scissors. Put the butter or margarine in a 1.25 litre/2¼ pt/5½ cup dish. Heat, uncovered, on Full for 1 minute. Add the onion. Cook, uncovered, on Full for 2 minutes, stirring once. Mix in all the remaining ingredients including the apricots. Use when cold.

Apple, Raisin and Walnut Stuffing

Makes 275 g/10 oz/12/3 cups

For pork, lamb, duck and goose.

25 g/1 oz/2 tbsp butter or margarine

1 eating (dessert) apple, peeled, quartered, cored and chopped

1 small onion, chopped

30 ml/2 tbsp raisins

30 ml/2 tbsp chopped walnuts

5 ml/1 tsp caster (superfine) sugar

125 g/4 oz/2 cups fresh white breadcrumbs

Salt and freshly ground black pepper

Put the butter or margarine in a 1.25 litre/2¼ pt/5½ cup dish. Heat, uncovered, on Full for 1 minute. Stir in the apple and onion. Cook, uncovered, on Full for 2 minutes, stirring once. Mix in all the remaining ingredients. Use when cold.

Apple, Prune and Brazil Nut Stuffing

Makes 275 g/10 oz/12/3 cups

For lamb and turkey.

Prepare as for Apple, Raisin and Walnut Stuffing, but substitute 8 stoned (pitted) and chopped prunes for the raisins and 30 ml/2 tbsp thinly sliced Brazil nuts for the walnuts.

Apple, Date and Hazelnut Stuffing

Makes 275 g/10 oz/12/3 cups

For lamb and game.

Prepare as for Apple, Raisin and Walnut Stuffing, but substitute 45 ml/3 tbsp chopped dates for the raisins and 30 ml/2 tbsp toasted and chopped hazelnuts for the walnuts.

Garlic, Rosemary and Lemon Stuffing

Makes 175 g/6 oz/1 cup

For lamb and pork.

25 g/1 oz/2 tbsp butter or margarine

2 garlic cloves, crushed

Grated peel of 1 small lemon

5 ml/1 tsp dried rosemary, crushed

15 ml/1 tbsp chopped parsley

125 g/4 oz/2 cups fresh white or brown breadcrumbs

Salt and freshly ground black pepper

Milk or dry red wine, if necessary

Put the butter or margarine in a 1 litre/1¾ pt/4¼ cup dish. Heat, uncovered, on Full for 1 minute. Stir in the garlic and lemon peel. Heat, uncovered, on Full for 30 seconds. Mix round and stir in the rosemary, parsley and breadcrumbs. Season to taste. Bind with milk or wine only if the stuffing remains on the dry side. Use when cold.

Garlic, Rosemary and Lemon Stuffing with Parmesan Cheese

Makes 175 g/6 oz/1 cup.

For beef.

Prepare as for Garlic, Rosemary and Lemon Stuffing, but add 45 ml/3 tbsp grated Parmesan cheese with the breadcrumbs.

Seafood Stuffing

Makes 275 g/10 oz/12/3 cups

For fish and vegetables.

25 g/1 oz/2 tbsp butter or margarine
125 g/4 oz/1 cup whole peeled prawns (shrimp)
5 ml/1 tsp finely grated lemon peel
125 g/4 oz/2 cups fresh white breadcrumbs
1 egg, beaten
Salt and freshly ground black pepper
Milk, if necessary

Put the butter or margarine in a 1 litre/1¾ pt/4¼ cup dish. Heat, uncovered, on Full for 1 minute. Stir in the prawns, lemon peel, breadcrumbs and egg and season to taste. Bind with milk only if the stuffing remains on the dry side. Use when cold.

Parma Ham Stuffing

Makes 275 g/10 oz/1⅔ cups

For poultry.

Prepare as for Seafood Stuffing, but substitute 75 g/3 oz/¾ cup coarsely chopped Parma ham for the prawns (shrimp).

Sausagemeat Stuffing

Makes 275 g/10 oz/1⅔ cups

For poultry and pork.

25 g/1 oz/2 tbsp butter or margarine
225 g/8 oz/1 cup pork or beef sausagemeat
1 small onion, grated
30 ml/2 tbsp finely chopped parsley
2.5 ml/½ tsp mustard powder
1 egg, beaten

Put the butter or margarine in a 1 litre/1¾ pt/4¼ cup dish. Heat, uncovered, on Full for 1 minute. Mix in the sausagemeat and onion. Cook, uncovered, on Full for 4 minutes, stirring every minute to ensure the sausagemeat is thoroughly broken up. Mix in all the remaining ingredients. Use when cold.

Sausagemeat and Liver Stuffing

Makes 275 g/10 oz/1 2/3 cups

For poultry.

Prepare as for Sausagemeat Stuffing, but reduce the sausagemeat to 175 g/6 oz/¾ cup. Add 50 g/2 oz/½ cup coarsely chopped chicken livers with the sausagemeat and onion.

Sausagemeat and Sweetcorn Stuffing

Makes 275 g/10 oz/1 2/3 cups

For poultry.

Prepare as for Sausagemeat Stuffing, but stir in 30–45 ml/2–3 tbsp cooked sweetcorn (corn) at the end of the cooking time.

Sausagemeat and Orange Stuffing

Makes 275 g/10 oz/1 2/3 cups

For poultry.

Prepare as for Sausagemeat Stuffing, but add 5–10 ml/1–2 tsp finely grated orange peel at the end of the cooking time

Chestnut Stuffing with Egg

Makes 350 g/12 oz/2 cups

For poultry.

125 g/4 oz/1 cup dried chestnuts, soaked overnight in water, then
drained
25 g/1 oz/2 tbsp butter or margarine
1 small onion, grated
1.5 ml/¼ tsp ground nutmeg
125 g/4 oz/2 cups fresh brown breadcrumbs
5 ml/1 tsp salt
1 large egg, beaten
15 ml/1 tbsp double (heavy) cream

Put the chestnuts in a 1.25 litre/2¼ pt/5½ cup casserole dish (Dutch oven) and cover with boiling water. Allow to stand for 5 minutes. Cover with clingfilm (plastic wrap) and slit it twice to allow steam to escape. Cook on Full for 30 minutes until the chestnuts are tender. Drain and allow to cool. Break up into small pieces. Put the butter or margarine in a 1.25 litre/2¼ pt/5½ cup dish. Heat, uncovered, on Full for 1 minute. Add the onion. Cook, uncovered, on Full for 2 minutes, stirring once. Mix in the chestnuts, nutmeg, breadcrumbs, salt and egg. Bind together with the cream. Use when cold.

Chestnut and Cranberry Stuffing

Makes 350 g/12 oz/2 cups

For poultry.

Prepare as for Chestnut Stuffing with Egg, but instead of egg, bind the stuffing with 30–45 ml/2–3 tbsp cranberry sauce. Add a little cream if the stuffing remains on the dry side.

Creamy Chestnut Stuffing

Makes 900 g/2 lb/5 cups

For poultry and fish.

50 g/2 oz/¼ cup butter, margarine or bacon dripping
1 onion, grated
500 g/1lb 2 oz/2¼ cups canned unsweetened chestnut purée
225 g/8 oz/4 cups fresh white breadcrumbs
Salt and freshly ground black pepper
2 eggs, beaten
Milk, if necessary

Put the butter, margarine or dripping in a 1¾ litre/3 pt/7½ cup dish. Heat, uncovered, on Full for 1½ minutes. Add the onion. Cook, uncovered, on Full for 2 minutes, stirring once. Thoroughly mix in the chestnut purée, breadcrumbs, salt and pepper to taste, and the eggs. Bind with milk only if the stuffing remains on the dry side. Use when cold.

Creamy Chestnut and Sausagement Stuffing

Makes 900 g/2 lb/5 cups

For poultry and game.

Prepare as for Creamy Chestnut Stuffing, but substitute 250 g/9 oz/generous 1 cup sausagemeat for half the chestnut purée.

Creamy Chestnut Stuffing with Whole Chestnuts

Makes 900 g/2 lb/5 cups

For poultry.

Prepare as for Creamy Chestnut Stuffing, but add 12 cooked and broken up chestnuts with the breadcrumbs.

Chestnut Stuffing with Parsley and Thyme

Makes 675 g/1½ lb/4 cups

For turkey and chicken.

15 ml/1 tbsp butter or margarine

5 ml/1 tsp sunflower oil

1 small onion, finely chopped

1 garlic clove, crushed

50 g/2 oz/1 cup parsley and thyme dry stuffing mix

440 g/15½ oz/2 cups canned unsweetened chestnut purée

150 ml/¼ pt/2/3 cup hot water

Finely grated peel of 1 lemon

1.5–2.5 ml/¼–½ tsp salt

Put the butter or margarine and oil in a 1.25 litre/2¼ pt/5½ cup bowl. Heat, uncovered, on Full for 25 seconds. Add the onion and garlic. Cook, uncovered, on Full for 3 minutes. Add the dry stuffing mix and stir in well. Cook, uncovered, on Full for 2 minutes, stirring twice. Remove from the microwave. Gradually stir in the chestnut purée alternately with the hot water until smoothly combined. Stir in the lemon peel and salt to taste. Use when cold.

Chestnut Stuffing with Gammon

Makes 675 g/1½ lb/4 cups

For turkey and chicken.

Prepare as for Chestnut Stuffing with Parsley and Thyme, but add 75 g/3 oz/¾ cup chopped gammon with the lemon peel and salt.

Chicken Liver Stuffing

Makes 350 g/12 oz/2 cups

For poultry and game.

125 g/4 oz/2/3 cup chicken livers
25 g/1 oz/2 tbsp butter or margarine
1 onion, grated
30 ml/2 tbsp finely chopped parsley
1.5 ml/¼ tsp ground allspice
125 g/4 oz/2 cups fresh white or brown breadcrumbs
Salt and freshly ground black pepper
Chicken stock, if necessary

Wash the livers and dry on kitchen paper. Cut into small pieces. Put the butter or margarine in a 1.25 litre/2¼ pt/5½ cup dish. Heat, uncovered, on Full for 1 minute. Add the onion. Cook, uncovered, on Full for 2 minutes, stirring once. Add the livers. Cook, uncovered, on Defrost for 3 minutes, stirring 3 times. Mix in the parsley, allspice and breadcrumbs and season to taste. Bind with a little stock only if the stuffing remains on the dry side. Use when cold.

Chicken Liver Stuffing with Pecans and Orange

Makes 350 g/12 oz/2 cups

For poultry and game.

Prepare as for Chicken Liver Stuffing, but add 30 ml/2 tbsp broken pecan nuts and 5 ml/1 tsp finely grated orange peel with the breadcrumbs.

Triple Nut Stuffing

Makes 350 g/12 oz/2 cups

For poultry and meat.

15 ml/1 tbsp sesame oil
1 garlic clove, crushed
125 g/4 oz/2/3 cup finely ground hazelnuts
125 g/4 oz/2/3 cup finely ground walnuts
125 g/4 oz/2/3 cup finely ground almonds
Salt and freshly ground black pepper
1 egg, beaten

Pour the oil into a fairly large dish. Heat, uncovered, on Full for 1 minute. Add the garlic. Cook, uncovered, on Full for 1 minute. Stir in all the nuts and season to taste. Bind with the egg. Use when cold.

Potato and Turkey Liver Stuffing

Makes 675 g/1½ lb/4 cups

For poultry.

450 g/1 lb floury potatoes
25 g/1 oz/2 tbsp butter or margarine
1 onion, chopped
2 rashers (slices) streaky bacon, chopped
5 ml/1 tsp dried mixed herbs
45 ml/3 tbsp finely chopped parsley
2.5 ml/½ tsp ground cinnamon
2.5 ml/½ tsp ground ginger
1 egg, beaten
Salt and freshly ground black pepper

Cook the potatoes as directed for Creamed Potatoes, but using only 60 ml/4 tbsp water. Drain and mash. Put the butter or margarine in a 1.25 litre/2¼ pt/5½ cup dish. Heat, uncovered, on Full for 1 minute. Stir in the onion and bacon. Cook, uncovered, on Full for 3 minutes, stirring twice. Mix in all the remaining ingredients including the potatoes, seasoning to taste. Use when cold.

Rice Stuffing with Herbs

Makes 450 g/1 lb/2⅔ cups

For poultry.

125 g/4 oz/⅔ cup easy-cook long-grain rice

250 ml/8 fl oz/1 cup boiling water

2.5 ml/½ tsp salt

25 g/1 oz/2 tbsp butter or margarine

1 small onion, grated

5 ml/1 tsp chopped parsley

5 ml/1 tsp coriander (cilantro) leaves

5 ml/1 tsp sage

5 ml/1 tsp basil leaves

Cook the rice with the water and salt as directed. Put the butter or margarine in a 1.25 litre/2¼ pt/5½ cup dish. Heat, uncovered, on Full for 1 minute. Stir in the onion. Cook, uncovered, on Full for 1 minute, stirring once. Mix in the rice and herbs. Use when cold.

Spanish Rice Stuffing with Tomato

Makes 450 g/1 lb/22/3 cups

For poultry.

125 g/4 oz/2/3 cup easy-cook long-grain rice
250 ml/8 fl oz/1 cup boiling water
2.5 ml/½ tsp salt
25 g/1 oz/2 tbsp butter or margarine
1 small onion, grated
30 ml/2 tbsp chopped green (bell) pepper
1 tomato, chopped
30 ml/2 tbsp chopped stuffed olives

Cook the rice with the water and salt as directed. Put the butter or margarine in a 1.25 litre/2¼ pt/5½ cup dish. Heat, uncovered, on Full for 1 minute. Stir in the onion, green pepper, tomato and olives. Cook, uncovered, on Full for 2 minute, stirring once. Mix in the rice. Use when cold.

Fruited Rice Stuffing

Makes 450 g/1 lb/2⅔ cups

For poultry.

125 g/4 oz/⅔ cup easy-cook long-grain rice

250 ml/8 fl oz/1 cup boiling water

2.5 ml/½ tsp salt

25 g/1 oz/2 tbsp butter or margarine

1 small onion, grated

5 ml/1 tsp chopped parsley

6 dried apricot halves, chopped

6 stoned (pitted) prunes, chopped

5 ml/1 tsp finely grated clementine or satsuma peel

Cook the rice with the water and salt as directed. Put the butter or margarine in a 1.25 litre/2¼ pt/5½ cup dish. Heat, uncovered, on Full for 1 minute. Stir in the onion, parsley, apricots, prunes and peel. Cook, uncovered, on Full for 1 minute, stirring once. Mix in the rice. Use when cold.

Far East Rice Stuffing

Makes 450 g/1 lb/22/3 cups

For poultry.

Prepare as for Rice Stuffing with Herbs, but use only the coriander (cilantro). Add 6 canned and sliced water chestnuts and 30 ml/2 tbsp coarsely chopped toasted cashew nuts with the onion.

Savoury Rice Stuffing with Nuts

Makes 450 g/1 lb/22/3 cups

For poultry.

Prepare as for Rice Stuffing with Herbs, but use only the parsley. Add 30 ml/2 tbsp flaked (slivered) and toasted almonds and 30 ml/2 tbsp salted peanuts with the onion.

Chocolate Crispies

Makes 16

75 g/3 oz/2/3 cup butter or margarine
30 ml/2 tbsp golden (light corn) syrup, melted
15 ml/1 tbsp cocoa (unsweetened chocolate) powder, sifted
45 ml/3 tbsp caster (superfine) sugar
75 g/3 oz/1½ cups cornflakes

Melt the butter or margarine and syrup, uncovered, on Defrost for 2–3 minutes. Stir in the cocoa and sugar. Fold in the cornflakes with a large metal spoon, tossing until well coated. Spoon into paper cake cases (cupcake papers), stand on a board or tray and chill until set.

Devil's Food Cake

Serves 8

A dream of a North American food processor cake, with a light and fluffy texture and deep chocolatey flavour.

100 g/4 oz/1 cup plain (semi-sweet) chocolate, broken into pieces
225 g/8 oz/2 cups self-raising (self-rising) flour
25 g/1 oz/2 tbsp cocoa (unsweetened chocolate) powder
1.5 ml/¼ tsp bicarbonate of soda (baking soda)
200 g/7 oz/scant 1 cup dark soft brown sugar
150 g/5 oz/2/3 cup butter or soft margarine, at kitchen temperature
5 ml/1 tsp vanilla essence (extract)
2 large eggs, at kitchen temperature
120 ml/4 fl oz/½ cup buttermilk or 60 ml/4 tbsp each skimmed milk and plain yoghurt
Icing (confectioners') sugar, for dusting

Closely line the base and sides of a straight-sided deep 20 cm/8 in diameter soufflé dish with clingfilm (plastic wrap). Melt the chocolate in a small bowl on Defrost for 3–4 minutes, stirring twice. Sift the flour, cocoa and bicarbonate of soda directly into a food processor bowl. Add the melted chocolate with all the remaining ingredients and process for about 1 minute or until the ingredients are well combined and the mixture resembles a thick batter. Spoon into the prepared dish and cover loosely with kitchen paper. Cook on Full for 9–10 minutes, turning the dish twice, until the cake has risen to the rim of the dish and the top is covered with small, broken bubbles and looks fairly dry. If any sticky patches remain, cook on Full for a further 20–30 seconds. Allow to stand in the microwave for about 15 minutes (the cake will fall slightly), then take it out and leave to cool until just warm. Carefully lift out of dish by holding the clingfilm and transfer to a wire rack to cool completely. Peel away the clingfilm and dust the top with sifted icing sugar before serving. Store in an airtight container.

Mocha Torte

Serves 8

Prepare as for Devil's Food Cake, but when cold cut the cake horizontally into three layers. Beat 450 ml/¾ pt/2 cups double (heavy) or whipping cream until thick. Sweeten to taste with a little sifted icing (confectioners') sugar, then flavour quite strongly with cold black coffee. Use some of the cream to sandwich the cake layers together, then swirl the remainder over the top and sides. Chill lightly before serving.

Multi-layer Cake

Serves 8

Prepare as for Devil's Food Cake, but when cold cut the cake horizontally into three layers. Sandwich together with apricot jam, whipped cream and grated chocolate or chocolate spread.

Black Forest Cherry Torte

Serves 8

Prepare as for Devil's Food Cake, but when cold cut the cake horizontally into three layers and moisten each with cherry liqueur. Sandwich together with cherry jam (conserve) or cherry fruit filling. Beat 300 ml/½ pt/1¼ cups double (heavy) or whipping cream until thick. Spread over the top and sides of the cake. Press a crushed chocolate flake bar or grated chocolate against the sides, then decorate the top with halved glacé (candied) cherries.

Chocolate Orange Gateau

Serves 8

Prepare as for Devil's Food Cake, but when cold cut the cake horizontally into three layers and moisten each with orange liqueur. Sandwich together with fine-shred orange marmalade and a thin round of marzipan (almond paste). Beat 300 ml/½ pt/1¼ cups double (heavy) or whipping cream until thick. Colour and sweeten lightly with 10–15 ml/2–3 tsp black treacle (molasses), then stir in 10 ml/2 tsp grated orange peel. Spread over the top and sides of the cake.

Chocolate Butter Cream Layer Cake

Serves 8–10

30 ml/2 tbsp cocoa (unsweetened chocolate) powder
60 ml/4 tbsp boiling water
175 g/6 oz/¾ cup butter or margarine, at kitchen temperature
175 g/6 oz/¾ cup dark soft brown sugar
5 ml/1 tsp vanilla essence (extract)
3 eggs, at kitchen temperature
175 g/6 oz/1½ cups self-raising (self-rising) flour
15 ml/1 tbsp black treacle (molasses)
Butter Cream Icing
Icing (confectioners') sugar, for dusting (optional)

Closely line the base and sides of an 18 x 9 cm/7 x 3½ in diameter soufflé dish with clingfilm (plastic wrap), allowing it to hang slightly over the edge. Mix the cocoa smoothly with the boiling water. Cream together the butter or margarine, sugar and vanilla essence until light and fluffy. Beat in the eggs one at a time, adding 15 ml/1 tbsp flour with each one. Fold in the remaining flour with the black treacle until evenly combined. Spread smoothly into the prepared dish and cover loosely with kitchen paper. Cook on Full for 6–6½ minutes until the cake is well risen and no longer damp- looking on top. Do not overcook or the cake will shrink and toughen. Allow to stand for 5 minutes, then ease the cake out of its dish by holding the clingfilm (plastic wrap) and transfer to a wire rack. Gently peel away the wrap and leave to cool. Cut the cake horizontally into three layers and sandwich together with the icing (frosting). Dust the top with sifted icing sugar before cutting, if liked.

Chocolate Mocha Cake

Serves 8–10

Prepare as for Chocolate Butter Cream Layer Cake, but flavour the Butter Cream Icing (frosting) with 15 ml/1 tbsp very strong black coffee. For a more intense flavour, add 5 ml/1 tsp ground coffee with the liquid coffee.

Orange-choc Layer Cake

Serves 8–10

Prepare as for Chocolate Butter Cream Layer Cake, but add 10 ml/2 tsp finely grated orange peel to the cake ingredients.

Double Chocolate Cake

Serves 8–10

Prepare as for Chocolate Butter Cream Layer Cake, but add 100 g/4 oz/1 cup melted and cooled plain (semi-sweet) chocolate to the Butter Cream Icing (frosting). Allow to firm up before using.

Whipped Cream and Walnut Torte

Serves 8–10

1 Chocolate Butter Cream Layer Cake
300 ml/½ pt/1¼ cups double (heavy) cream
150 ml/¼ pt/2/3 cup whipping cream
45 ml/3 tbsp icing (confectioners') sugar, sifted
Any flavouring essence (extract), such as vanilla, rose, coffee, lemon,
orange, almond, ratafia
Nuts, chocolate shavings, silver dragees, crystallised flower petals or
glacé (candied) fruits, to decorate

Cut the cake horizontally into three layers. Beat together the creams until thick. Fold in the icing sugar and flavouring to taste. Sandwich the cake layers together with the cream and decorate the top as wished.

Christmas Gâteau

Serves 8–10

1 Chocolate Butter Cream Layer Cake
45 ml/3 tbsp seedless raspberry jam (conserve)
Marzipan (almond paste)
300 ml/½ pt/1¼ cups double (heavy) cream
150 ml/¼ pt/2/3 cup whipping cream
60 ml/4 tbsp caster (superfine) sugar
Glacé (candied) cherries and edible holly sprigs, to decorate

Cut the cake into three layers and sandwich together with the jam topped with thinly rolled out rounds of marzipan. Beat together the creams and caster sugar until thick and use to cover the top and sides of the cake. Decorate the top with cherries and holly.

American Brownies

Makes 12

50 g/2 oz/½ cup plain (semi-sweet) chocolate, broken into pieces

75 g/3 oz/2/3 cup butter or margarine

175 g/6 oz/¾ cup dark soft brown sugar

2 eggs, at kitchen temperature, beaten

150 g/5 oz/1¼ cups plain (all-purpose) flour

1.5 ml/¼ tsp baking powder

5 ml/1 tsp vanilla essence (extract)

30 ml/2 tbsp cold milk

Icing (confectioners') sugar, for dusting

Butter and base line a 25 x 16 3 5 cm/10 x 6½ 3 2 in dish. Melt the chocolate and butter or margarine on Full for 2 minutes, stirring until well mixed. Beat in the sugar and eggs until well combined. Sift together the flour and baking powder, then lightly stir into the chocolate mixture with the vanilla essence and milk. Spread evenly into the prepared dish and cover loosely with kitchen paper. Cook on Full for 7 minutes until the cake is well risen and the top is peppered with small broken air holes. Allow to cool in the dish for 10 minutes. Cut into squares, dust the tops fairly thickly with icing sugar, then leave to cool completely on a wire rack. Store in an airtight container.

Chocolate Nut Brownies

Makes 12

Prepare as for American Brownies, but add 90 ml/6 tbsp coarsely chopped walnuts with the sugar. Cook for 1 minute extra.

Oaten Toffee Triangles

Makes 8

125 g/4 oz/½ cup butter or margarine

50 g/2 oz/3 tbsp golden (light corn) syrup

25 ml/1½ tbsp black treacle (molasses)

100 g/4 oz/½ cup dark soft brown sugar

225 g/8 oz/2 cups porridge oats

Thoroughly grease a deep 20 cm/8 in diameter dish. Melt together the butter, syrup, treacle and sugar, uncovered, on Defrost for 5 minutes. Stir in the oats and spread the mixture into the dish. Cook, uncovered, on Full for 4 minutes, turning the dish once. Allow to stand for 3 minutes. Cook for a further 1½ minutes. Allow to cool to lukewarm, then cut into eight triangles. Remove from the dish when cold and store in an airtight container.

Muesli Triangles

Makes 8

Prepare as for Oaten Toffee Triangles, but substitute unsweetened muesli for the porridge oats.

Chocolate Queenies

Makes 12

125 g/4 oz/1 cup self-raising (self-rising) flour
30 ml/2 tbsp cocoa (unsweetened chocolate) powder
50 g/2 oz/¼ cup butter or margarine, at kitchen temperature
50 g/2 oz/¼ cup light soft brown sugar
1 egg
5 ml/1 tsp vanilla essence (extract)
30 ml/2 tbsp cold milk
Icing (confectioners') sugar or chocolate spread, to decorate
(optional)

Sift together the flour and cocoa. In a separate bowl, cream together the butter or margarine and sugar until soft and fluffy. Beat in the egg and vanilla essence. Fold in the flour mixture alternately with the milk, stirring briskly with a fork without beating. Divide between 12 paper cake cases (cupcake papers). Place six at a time on the glass or plastic turntable, cover loosely with kitchen paper and cook on Full for 2 minutes. Cool on a wire rack. Dust with sifted icing sugar or cover with chocolate spread, if wished. Store in an airtight container.

Flaky Chocolate Queenies

Makes 12

Prepare as for Chocolate Queenies, but crush a small chocolate flake bar and gently stir it into the cake mixture after the egg and vanilla essence have been added.

Breakfast Bran and Pineapple Cake

Makes about 12 pieces

A fairly dense cake and a useful snack breakfast served with yoghurt and a drink.

100 g/3½ oz/1 cup All Bran cereal

50 g/2 oz/¼ cup dark soft brown sugar

175 g/6 oz canned crushed pineapple

20 ml/4 tsp thick honey

1 egg, beaten

300 ml/½ pt/1¼ cups skimmed milk

150 g/5 oz/1¼ cups self-raising (self-rising) wholemeal flour

Closely line the base and sides of an 18 cm/7 in diameter soufflé dish with clingfilm (plastic wrap), allowing it to hang very slightly over the edge. Put the cereal, sugar, pineapple and honey into a bowl. Cover with a plate and warm on Defrost for 5 minutes. Mix in the remaining ingredients, stirring briskly without beating. Transfer to the prepared dish. Cover loosely with kitchen paper and cook on Defrost for 20 minutes, turning the dish four times. Leave until cooled to just warm, then transfer to a wire rack by holding the clingfilm. When completely cold, store in an airtight container for 1 day before cutting.

Fruited Chocolate Biscuit Crunch Cake

Makes 10–12

200 g/7 oz/scant 1 cup plain (semi-sweet) chocolate, broken into squares

225 g/8 oz/1 cup unsalted (sweet) butter (not margarine)

2 large eggs, at kitchen temperature, beaten

5 ml/1 tsp vanilla essence (extract)

75 g/3 oz/¾ cup coarsely chopped mixed nuts

75 g/3 oz/¾ cup chopped crystallised pineapple or papaya

75 g/3 oz/¾ cup chopped crystallised ginger

25 ml/1½ tbsp icing (confectioners') sugar, sifted

15 ml/1 tbsp fruit liqueur, such as Grand Marnier or Cointreau

225 g/8 oz plain sweet biscuits (cookies) such as digestives (Graham crackers), each snapped into 8 pieces

Closely line the base and sides of a 20 cm/8 in diameter dish or sponge sandwich tin (pan) with clingfilm (plastic wrap). Melt the chocolate pieces in a large bowl, uncovered, on Defrost for 4–5 minutes until very soft but still holding their original shape. Cut the butter into large cubes and melt, uncovered, on Defrost for 2–3 minutes. Stir thoroughly into the melted chocolate with the eggs and vanilla essence. Mix in all the remaining ingredients. When well combined, spread into the prepared tin and cover with foil or clingfilm (plastic wrap). Chill for 24 hours, then carefully lift out and peel away the clingfilm. Cut into wedges to serve. Keep refrigerated between servings as the cake softens at room temperature.

Fruited Mocha Biscuit Crunch Cake

Makes 10–12

Prepare as for Fruited Chocolate Biscuit Crunch Cake, but melt 20 ml/4 tsp instant coffee powder or granules with the chocolate and substitute coffee liqueur for the fruit liqueur.

Fruited Rum and Raisin Biscuit Crunch Cake

Makes 10–12

Prepare as for Fruited Chocolate Biscuit Crunch Cake, but substitute 100 g/3½ oz/¾ cup raisins for the crystallised fruit and substitute dark rum for the liqueur.

Fruited Whisky and Orange Biscuit Crunch Cake

Makes 10–12

Prepare as for Fruited Chocolate Biscuit Crunch Cake, but stir the finely grated peel of 1 orange into the chocolate and butter and substitute whisky for the liqueur.

White Chocolate Fruited Crunch Cake

Makes 10–12

Prepare as for Fruited Chocolate Biscuit Crunch Cake, but substitute white chocolate for dark.

Two-layer Apricot and Raspberry Cheesecake

Serves 12

For the base:
100 g/3½ oz/½ cup butter
225 g/8 oz/2 cups chocolate digestive biscuit (Graham cracker) crumbs
5 ml/1 tsp mixed (apple-pie) spice

For the apricot layer:
60 ml/4 tbsp cold water
30 ml/2 tbsp powdered gelatine
500 g/1 lb 2 oz/2¼ cups curd (smooth cottage) cheese
250 g/9 oz/1¼ cups fromage frais or quark
60 ml/4 tbsp smooth apricot jam (conserve)
75 g/3 oz/2/3 cup caster (superfine) sugar
3 eggs, separated
A pinch of salt

For the raspberry layer:
45 ml/3 tbsp cold water

15 ml/1 tbsp powdered gelatine

225 g/8 oz fresh raspberries, crushed and sieved (strained)

30 ml/2 tbsp caster (superfine) sugar

150 ml/¼ pt/2/3 cup double (heavy) cream

For decoration:

Fresh raspberries, strawberries and strings of redcurrants

To make the base, melt the butter, uncovered, on Defrost for 3–3½ minutes. Stir in the biscuit crumbs and mixed spice. Spread evenly over the base of a 25 cm/10 in diameter springform cake tin (pan). Chill for 30 minutes until firm.

To make the apricot layer, put the water and gelatine into a basin and stir well to mix. Stand for 5 minutes until softened. Melt, uncovered, on Defrost for 2½–3 minutes. Put in a food processor with the curd cheese, fromage frais or quark, jam, sugar and egg yolks and run the machine until the ingredients are thoroughly combined. Scrape out into a large bowl, cover with a plate and chill until just beginning to thicken and set round the edge. Whisk the egg whites and salt to stiff peaks. Beat one-third into the cheese mixture, then fold in the remainder with a metal spoon or spatula. Spread evenly over the biscuit base. Cover loosely with kitchen paper and chill for at least 1 hour until firm.

To make the raspberry layer, put the water and gelatine into a basin and stir well to mix. Stand for 5 minutes until softened. Melt, uncovered, on Defrost for 1½–2 minutes. Combine with the raspberry purée and sugar. Cover with foil or clingfilm (plastic wrap) and chill until just beginning to thicken and set round the edge. Beat the cream until softly thickened. Beat one-third into the fruit mixture, then fold in the remainder with a metal spoon or spatula. Spread evenly over the cheesecake mixture. Cover loosely and chill for several hours until firm. To serve, run a knife dipped in hot water round the inside edge to loosen the cheesecake. Unclip the tin and remove the side. Decorate the top with fruits. Cut into portions with a knife dipped in hot water.

Peanut Butter Cheesecake

Serves 10

For the base:
100 g/3½ oz/½ cup butter
225 g/8 oz/2 cups ginger biscuit (cookie) crumbs

For the topping:
90 ml/6 tbsp cold water
45 ml/3 tbsp powdered gelatine
750 g/1½ lb/3 cups curd (smooth cottage) cheese
4 eggs, separated
5 ml/1 tsp vanilla essence (extract)
150 g/5 oz/2/3 cup caster (superfine) sugar
A pinch of salt
150 ml/¼ pt/2/3 cup double (heavy) cream
60 ml/4 tbsp smooth peanut butter, at kitchen temperature
Chopped lightly salted or plain peanuts (optional)

To make the base, melt the butter, uncovered, on Defrost for 3–3½ minutes. Stir in the biscuit crumbs. Spread over the base of a 20 cm/8 in diameter springform tin (pan) and chill for 20–30 minutes until firm.

To make the topping, put the water and gelatine into a basin and stir well to mix. Stand for 5 minutes to soften. Melt, uncovered, on Defrost for 3–3½ minutes. Put in a food processor with the cheese, egg yolks, vanilla essence and sugar and run the machine until smooth. Scrape out into a large bowl. Whisk the egg whites and salt to stiff peaks. Whip the cream until softly thickened. Fold the egg whites and cream alternately into the cheese mixture. Finally, swirl in the peanut butter. Spread evenly into the prepared tin, cover securely and chill for at least 12 hours. To serve, run a knife dipped in hot water round the side to loosen. Unclip the tin and remove the sides. Decorate with chopped peanuts, if liked. Cut into portions with a knife dipped in hot water.

Lemon Curd Cheesecake

Serves 10

Prepare as for Peanut Butter Cheesecake, but substitute lemon curd for the peanut butter.

Chocolate Cheesecake

Serves 10

Prepare as for Peanut Butter Cheesecake, but substitute chocolate spread for the peanut butter.

Sharon Fruit Cheesecake

Serves 10

A recipe, sent to me by a New Zealand lady, based on the tomato-like fruit tamarillo. As they are not always easy to obtain, winter sharon fruit make an admirable substitute, or even the look-alike persimmon as long as they are very ripe.

For the base:

175 g/6 oz/¾ cup butter

100 g/3½ oz/½ cup light soft brown sugar

225 g/8 oz malt biscuit (cookie) crumbs

For the filling:

4 sharon fruit, chopped

100 g/4 oz/½ cup light soft brown sugar

30 ml/2 tbsp powdered gelatine

30 ml/2 tbsp cold water

300 g/10 oz/1¼ cups cream cheese

3 large eggs, separated

Juice of ½ lemon

Thoroughly rinse a 25 cm/10 in diameter springform tin (pan) and leave wet. Melt the butter or margarine, uncovered, on Defrost for 3–3½ minutes. Stir in the sugar and biscuit crumbs. Press evenly over the base of the tin. Chill while preparing the cake filling.

To make the filling, put the sharon fruit into a dish and sprinkle with half the sugar. Put the gelatine into a basin and stir in the water. Stand for 5 minutes until softened. Melt, uncovered, on Defrost for 3–3½ minutes. In separate bowl, beat the cheese until soft and fluffy, then work in the gelatine, egg yolks, lemon juice and remaining sugar. Whisk the egg whites to stiff peaks. Fold into the cheese mixture alternatively with the sharon fruit. Spoon over the biscuit base and chill overnight. To serve, run a knife dipped in hot water round the side to loosen, then unclip the tin and remove the sides.

Blueberry Cheesecake

Serves 10

Prepare as for Sharon Fruit Cheesecake, but substitute 350 g/12 oz blueberries for the sharon fruit.

Baked Lemon Cheesecake

Serves 10

For the base:

75 g/3 oz/1/3 cup butter, at kitchen temperature

175 g/6 oz/1½ cups digestive biscuit (Graham cracker) crumbs

30 ml/2 tbsp caster (superfine) sugar

For the filling:

450 g/1 lb/2 cups medium-fat curd (smooth cottage) cheese, at kitchen

temperature

75 g/3 oz/1/3 cup caster (superfine) sugar

2 large eggs, at kitchen temperature

5 ml/1 tsp vanilla essence (extract)

15 ml/1 tbsp cornflour (cornstarch)

Finely grated peel and juice of 1 lemon

150 ml/¼ pt/2/3 cup double (heavy) cream

150 ml/5 oz/2/3 cup soured (dairy sour) cream

To make the base, melt the butter, uncovered, on Defrost for 2–2½ minutes. Stir in the biscuit crumbs and sugar. Line the base and side of a 20 cm/8 in diameter dish with clingfilm (plastic wrap), allowing it to hang very slightly over the edge. Cover the base and sides with the biscuit mixture. Cook, uncovered, on Full for 2½ minutes.

To make the filling, beat the cheese until soft, then blend in the remaining ingredients except the soured cream. Pour into the crumb

214

case and cover loosely with kitchen paper. Cook on Full for 12 minutes, turning the dish twice. The cake is ready when there is some movement to be seen in the middle and the top has risen slightly and is just beginning to crack. Allow to stand for 5 minutes. Remove from the microwave and gently spread with the soured cream, which will set on top and even out as the cake cools.

Baked Lime Cheesecake

Serves 10

Prepare as for Baked Lemon Cheesecake, but substitute the peel and juice of 1 lime for the lemon.

Baked Blackcurrant Cheesecake

Serves 10

Prepare as for Baked Lemon Cheesecake, but when completely cold spread the top with either good-quality blackcurrant jam (conserve) or canned blackcurrant fruit filling.

Baked Raspberry Cheesecake

Serves 10

Prepare as for Baked Lemon Cheesecake, but substitute raspberry blancmange powder for the cornflour (cornstarch). Decorate the top with fresh raspberries.

Green Tomato Chutney

Makes 900 g/2 lb

Prepare as for Apple Chutney, but substitute coarsely chopped green tomatoes for the apples.

Banana and Green Pepper Chutney

Makes 900 g/2 lb

Prepare as for Apple Chutney, but substitute bananas for the apples and add a finely chopped seeded green (bell) pepper with all the remaining ingredients.

Dark Plum Chutney

Makes 900 g/2 lb

Prepare as for Apple Chutney, but substitute stoned (pitted) plums for the apples and add 1 star anise to the pickling spice for a slightly oriental flavour.

Bread and Butter Pickles

Makes 750 g/1½ lb

A North American clear relish, slightly on the sweet side, with a distinctive personality and a brilliant golden hue from the turmeric. It goes beautifully with cold meats and hamburgers, cheese, poultry and fried fish but does best in sandwiches.

1 large cucumber (about 450 g/1 lb), unpeeled and cut into paper-thin slices

2 large onions, peeled and cut into paper-thin slices

175 ml/6 fl oz/¾ cup colourless distilled malt vinegar

175 g/6 oz/¾ cup caster (superfine) sugar

10 ml/2 tsp mixed pickling spice

10 ml/2 tsp salt

1.5 ml/¼ tsp mustard powder

1.5 ml/¼ tsp turmeric

4–5 sprays dill (dill weed)

Put the cucumber and onion slices in a colander (strainer) and leave to stand for 30 minutes to drain. Meanwhile, pour the vinegar into a 2 litre/3½ pt/8½ cup bowl. Stir in the sugar, pickling spice, salt, mustard and turmeric. Heat, uncovered, on Full for 5 minutes, stirring twice. Mix in the cucumber, onions and dill. Heat, uncovered, on Full for 3 minutes, stirring twice. Allow to cool to lukewarm, then transfer to one large or two medium jam (conserve) jars. Cover when cold and store in the refrigerator.

FILLED CROISSANTS

The following recipes contain some delicious ideas with croissants.

Cream Cheese and Pickle

1 croissant

30 ml/2 tbsp full-cream or low-fat cream cheese

15 ml/1 tbsp sweet pickle

1 small tomato, thinly sliced

Halve the croissant and spread the cut sides with cheese. Sandwich together with pickle and tomato. Put on a plate and heat, uncovered, on Defrost for 30–35 seconds until warm.

Ham Mayonnaise with Salad

1 croissant

15 ml/1 tbsp mild wholegrain mustard

2 thin slices ham

15 ml/1 tbsp mayonnaise

1 small sliced cooked beetroot (red beet)

Halve the croissant and spread the cut sides with mustard. Sandwich together with the remaining ingredients. Put on a plate and heat, uncovered, on Defrost for 30–35 seconds until warm.

Turkey and Coleslaw

1 croissant

Butter or margarine

2 slices cold turkey from a roast bird or a packet

30 ml/2 tbsp coleslaw

Halve the croissant and spread the cut sides with butter or margarine. Sandwich together with the remaining ingredients. Put on a plate and heat, uncovered, on Defrost for 35–40 seconds until warm.

Savoury Peanut Butter and Lettuce

1 croissant

Smooth peanut butter

Yeast extract

Soft lettuce leaves

Halve the croissant and spread the cut sides with peanut butter followed by yeast extract. Sandwich together with 2 or 3 lettuce leaves. Put on a plate and heat, uncovered, on Defrost for 20–25 seconds until warm.

CPSIA information can be obtained
at www.ICGtesting.com
Printed in the USA
LVHW040149131222
735056LV00002B/191